the RITALIN
FACT BOOK

BOOKS BY PETER R. BREGGIN, M.D.

Nonfiction

College Students in a Mental Hospital: An Account of Organized Social Contacts Between College Volunteers and Mental Patients in a Hospital Community (1962) (Jointly authored with Umbarger et al.)

Electroshock: Its Brain-Disabling Effects (1979)

The Psychology of Freedom: Liberty and Love as a Way of Life (1980)

Psychiatric Drugs: Hazards to the Brain (1983)

Toxic Psychiatry: Why Therapy, Empathy and Love Must Replace the Drugs, Electroshock and Biochemical Theories of the "New Psychiatry" (1991)

Beyond Conflict: From Self-Help and Psychotherapy to Peacemaking (1992)

Talking Back to Prozac: What Doctors Aren't Telling You About Today's Most Controversial Drug (1994) (Coauthored by Ginger Ross Breggin)

Psychosocial Approaches to Deeply Disturbed Persons (1996) (Coedited by E. Mark Stern)

Brain-Disabling Treatments in Psychiatry: Drugs, Electroshock and the Role of the FDA (1997)

The Heart of Being Helpful: Empathy and the Creation of a Healing Presence (1997)

The War Against Children of Color: Psychiatry Targets Inner-City Youth (1998) (Coauthored by Ginger Ross Breggin)

Talking Back to Ritalin: What Doctors Aren't Telling You About Stimulants for Children (1998)

Your Drug May Be Your Problem: How and Why to Stop Taking Psychiatric Medications (1999) (Coauthored by David Cohen)

Reclaiming Our Children: A Healing Solution for a Nation in Crisis (2000)

Talking Back to Ritalin Revised Edition (2001)

The Antidepressant Fact Book (2001)

Dimensions of Empathic Therapy (2002) (Coauthored by Ginger Breggin and Fred Bemak)

Fiction

The Crazy from the Sane (1971)

After the Good War (1972)

the RITALIN FACT BOOK

WHAT YOUR DOCTOR WON'T TELL YOU ABOUT ADHD AND STIMULANT DRUGS

PETER R. BREGGIN, M.D.

PERSEUS
PUBLISHING

A Member of the Perseus Books Group

Library of Congress Control Number: 2002105973
ISBN 0-7382-0450-1

Perseus Publishing is a member of the Perseus Books Group.
Find us on the World Wide Web at http://www.perseuspublishing.com.

Perseus Publishing books are available at special discounts for bulk purchases in the U.S. by corporations, institutions, and other organizations. For more information, please contact the Special Markets Department at the Perseus Books Group, 11 Cambridge Center, Cambridge, MA 02142, or call (800) 255-1514 or (617) 252-5298, or e-mail j.mccrary@perseusbooks.com.

Text design by *Reginald Thompson*
Set in 10.5-point Sabon by the Perseus Books Group

First printing, July 2002

1 2 3 4 5 6 7 8 9 10—04 03 02

For my wife, Ginger Breggin—
Nineteen years and more than a dozen books later,
She continues to inspire me.

Contents

List of Tables   *ix*

Acknowledgments   *xi*

The Stimulant Drugs   *xiii*

Be Informed   *xv*

Introduction: Facts Unavailable Anywhere Else   *xvii*

Part I: Understanding Stimulant Medication   **1**

Chapter 1: A Factual Antidote to Stimulant
   Drug Misinformation   2

Chapter 2: A Child's Journey Through Psychiatric
   Diagnoses and Drugs   4

Chapter 3: Of Cages and Creativity—How Stimulants Work   16

Chapter 4: How Stimulants Cause Psychiatric Disorders   30

Chapter 5: How Stimulants Harm the Child's Brain   43

Chapter 6: How Stimulants Harm the Child's Body   53

Chapter 7: How Stimulants Cause Withdrawal,
   Addiction, and Abuse   67

Chapter 8: How to Withdraw from Stimulants   77

Chapter 9: Do Stimulants Really Help with "ADHD"?   85

Chapter 10: Do Antidepressants and Other Drugs
   Help with "ADHD"?   92

Chapter 11: Do "Alternative Treatments"
   Help with "ADHD"?   107

Chapter 12: The Ultimate Source of Misinformation   112

Part II: Understanding and Improving ADHD-Like Behaviors 121

Chapter 13: The Real Nature of "ADHD" 122

Chapter 14: The Real Nature of "Learning Disorders" 137

Chapter 15: Why "ADHD" Should Not Be
Considered a Disability 147

Chapter 16: How to Provide Guidance in the Family 152

Chapter 17: How to Help Out-of-Control Children 161

Chapter 18: How to Provide Guidance in
the Classroom and Other Groups 175

Chapter 19: When the School Says Your Child Has a Problem 189

Chapter 20: Getting Worse Before It Gets Better 195

Chapter 21: After September 11—A Better Future
for Our Children 201

Notes 205

Bibliography 215

Index 225

About the Author 235

List of Tables

Tables

3.1 *Harmful stimulant drug reactions commonly
    misidentified as "therapeutic" or "beneficial"*   24

4.1 *Toxic reactions to stimulants: Usually in overdose
    and occasionally at low doses*   32
4.2 *Overview of harmful reactions to stimulant drugs:
    Ritalin, Dexedrine, Adderall, Concerta, and Metadate*   33
4.3 *Rates of adverse mental effects reported in
    stimulant clinical trials*   35

5.1 *Stimulant-induced brain damage and dysfunction
    demonstrated in human and animal research*   44

13.1 *Diagnostic criteria for Attention-Deficit/
    Hyperactivity Disorder*   127

Acknowledgments

I am feeling the need to write an entire book to communicate what my wife, Ginger Breggin, means to me personally and to my work. In the meantime, let me simply say that for nearly twenty years, Ginger has inspired, guided, educated, and loved me on a daily basis and at critical moments in our lives. Thank you again.

I also want to thank again her mom and dad, Jean and Phil Ross. Jean, a former schoolteacher, made a special contribution to this book.

My research assistant, Ian Goddard, was better than ever and provided help at every stage of the book from its inception to its editing.

Finally, I want to thank David Cohen, Ph.D.; Milton Shore, Ph.D.; and Kevin McCready, Ph.D., for helping to edit and comment on this manuscript. It was very generous of them to take time from their busy professional careers.

Once again, I want especially to recognize the work of Dr. Kevin McCready, the founder and director of the San Joaquin Psychotherapy Center in Clovis, California, who continues to provide the profession with a model of how to run a drug-free mental health clinic based on sound ethical and therapeutic values. For those interested in this approach to helping people, the International Center for the Study of Psychiatry and Psychology welcomes you to participate in its activities. I am in the process of handing over the leadership to younger professionals and look forward to watching them bring new zeal to the projects. In the meantime, the center can be contacted through my web site, www.breggin.com.

The Stimulant Drugs

Four to six million children and many additional adults are now taking central nervous system stimulant drugs for "attention deficit hyperactivity disorder" (ADHD) and similar problems. These drugs include the following:

Shorter-Acting Stimulants:

> Ritalin, Methylin (methylphenidate)
> Focalin (d-methylphenidate)
> Dexedrine, Dextrostat (d-amphetamine)
> Adderall (amphetamine mixture)
> Desoxyn (methamphetamine)
> Cylert (pemoline)

Longer-Acting Stimulants:

> Concerta, Metadate ER, Ritalin SR, Ritalin LA, Methylin
> ER (methylphenidate)
> Adderall XR (amphetamine mixture)

The longer-acting forms are sustained-release preparations. The chemicals are unchanged but are released more slowly into the bloodstream.

Be Informed

All of the commonly prescribed stimulants for ADHD are either amphetamines or amphetamine-like and share common effects and hazards. Adderall and Dexedrine are amphetamines and Ritalin, Focalin, and Concerta are amphetamine-like. Cylert, or pemoline, is an exception, but it is rarely used in the United States and has been withdrawn in Canada because of special hazards, including potentially fatal liver disease.

All the commonly used stimulants are highly addictive and subject to abuse. All are similar to cocaine in their properties. They can cause many physical problems, including cardiovascular dysfunction, growth suppression, and tics. They can also cause many serious psychiatric side effects such as agitation, aggression, psychosis, mania, depression, and obsessive-compulsive disorder.

Stimulant drugs can cause withdrawal symptoms. For days, weeks, or even longer after stopping them, the brain struggles to regain its normal chemical balance. Animal studies indicate that the brain does not always fully recover from routine clinical doses.

Abrupt stimulant withdrawal can produce potentially life-threatening reactions, including fatigue, depression, and suicidality. Especially if the drugs have been used for prolonged periods of time, they should be stopped slowly with gradually reduced doses under the supervision of an experienced clinician.

This book is written from a viewpoint that is critical of stimulant drugs and their prescription for "attention deficit hyperactivity disorder." There are, of course, innumerable other books that provide a much more favorable picture, including the *Physicians' Desk Reference (PDR)*, an annual publication readily available in bookstores, libraries, and on the Web at www.pdr.net. The *PDR* contains the official drug label (package insert) as approved by the Food and Drug Administration (FDA).

No book, critical or promotional, can substitute for informed clinical evaluations, including second opinions from experts. Educate yourself, become informed, and make up your own mind before taking stimulants for ADHD or giving them to your child.

Introduction: Facts Unavailable Anywhere Else

Many of the facts presented in this book concerning Ritalin, Focalin,[1] Adderall, Concerta, and other stimulants are unavailable from the usual sources, such as popular books and professional articles and textbooks. Many are unknown to a significant percentage of medical doctors who prescribe the drugs. My own knowledge derives from many sources, including more than three decades of full-time psychiatric practice working with adults and with children, families, and schools. As a part of my clinical work as a physician, I am frequently consulted as a "doctor of last resort" on behalf of children and adults who have been harmed by stimulant drugs.

As a psychiatrist, I never start children or adults on psychiatric medications, including stimulants. I advocate the psychosocial school of psychiatry that emphasizes the value of psychotherapy, family therapy, educational improvements, and other human services over the use of drugs. When a child has a problem in the home or at school, I work with the significant adults in the child's life, including parents and teachers. Often most of the therapeutic work is done with the adults, who then make the necessary changes to address the child's needs.

Although I avoid starting children or adults on psychiatric medication, I have a great deal of experience in prescribing drugs and evaluating their effects. Patients often come to me for help in withdrawing from psychiatric medication, and during the process I may have to prescribe the drugs for many months. Other patients feel unable to completely stop their medications because they have become physically and psychologically dependent on them. They want my help in maintaining the lowest possible dose. Many patients also come to me for help in understanding and recovering from the harm that has been done to them by psychiatric medications. I frequently have to prescribe or evaluate the effects of complex combinations of psychiatric drugs that have been administered for many years.

In addition to my more than three decades of clinical work, this book also draws upon the years of research required for writing dozens of scientific books and articles; the workshops I have given for professionals and the public; teaching I have done in the past at universities, including the Johns Hopkins University Department of Counseling; and presentations I have made at national conferences for health professionals and attorneys.

In November 1998, for example, I was asked by the National Institutes of Health (NIH) to be the scientific presenter on the "Risks and Mechanism of Action of Stimulants" at the government's national Consensus Development Conference on the Diagnosis and Treatment of Attention Deficit Hyperactivity Disorder. In September 2000, I was asked to give testimony concerning "Behavioral Drugs in Schools: Questions and Concerns" before the Committee on Education and the Workforce of the U.S. House of Representatives. In May 2001, I spoke by invitation on "The Science and Medicine of Ritalin" at a conference on Emerging Drug Litigation Strategies organized by Mealey's (Lexis/Nexis) in New Orleans for attorneys.

I am founder and director of the International Center for the Study of Psychiatry and Psychology (ICSPP), an organization of 2,000 reform-minded professionals in the field of mental health. The center sponsors a peer-reviewed scientific journal and holds international conferences that often deal with drug-related issues.

It also receives daily inquiries and informative communications from professionals, media representatives, lawyers, and consumers from around the world. As a result, I often hear about newly discovered adverse drug reactions long before most professionals become aware of them.

The International Center for the Study of Psychiatry and Psychology carries on many reform activities in the professional and public arenas and is the leading professional organization in challenging the increasing drugging of America's children.

I have yet another unique source of information and knowledge. For many years I have been a consultant and medical expert in legal actions involving psychiatric drugs, including the stimulants described in this book. I have researched and written innumerable reports and testified in court cases, often concerning stimulants and ADHD. Some cases involve parents who are being pressured to give stimulants to their children. Others involve children and adults who have been injured by the drugs. Most dramatically, I've been an expert in criminal cases in which Ritalin, Adderall, and other stimulants have played a role in making children or adults psychotic and violent or have led to cocaine addiction and crime.

My most specialized source of information about psychiatric drugs comes from my work as a medical expert in cases against giant pharmaceutical companies that are charged with negligence or fraud in developing or publicizing their products. In this fascinating legal arena, I can gain access to secret "inside information" about psychiatric medications that is literally unavailable to any other physician in the world. In some cases, I spend several days inside the drug companies themselves examining their records on drug testing and promotion. Beyond gaining unique inside information, these experiences have honed my scientific acumen.

Based on my publications and consultations, a series of class-action suits have been brought against Novartis, the manufacturer of Ritalin, charging the company with conspiring with the

American Psychiatric Association and the parents' group Children and Adults with Attention Deficit Disorder (CHADD) to fabricate the ADHD diagnosis and to foster the overuse of Ritalin.

In addition to examining the limitations and potential dangers of stimulant drugs, *The Ritalin Fact Book* will also examine the ADHD diagnosis and how it is misused to justify prescribing these drugs. Then it will provide better approaches to helping children and adults with ADHD-like behaviors or problems.

This is a book of facts. Above all else, it aims to provide adults with the kind of information they need to make responsible decisions about taking stimulant medications or giving them to the children in their care.

PART I

Understanding Stimulant Medication

A Factual Antidote to Stimulant Drug Misinformation

Have you seen the multicolor ads in *Good Housekeeping, Ladies' Home Journal,* and other national magazines? One shows two little children giggling together in delight, supposedly because they are taking stimulant drugs. Another shows a mother holding her child in a warm embrace while they smile, again because the child takes a stimulant drug.

Or have you read some of the many books and magazine articles or visited web sites touting the use of pharmaceutical agents for controlling or improving the behavior of children?

Or has a pediatrician, family doctor, neurologist, or psychiatrist recommended stimulants such as Ritalin, Concerta, Focalin, or Adderall for you or for your child?

Or do you have a grandchild or other family member who is taking these medications?

This book is a *factual antidote* to the stimulant-drug advertising, promotion, and misinformation that is deluging the nation and much of the Western world. It is meant for anyone who cares about the millions of children and adults who are being diagnosed with attention deficit hyperactivity disorder (ADHD) and are being prescribed stimulant drugs such as Ritalin, Focalin,

Adderall, and Dexedrine and long-acting preparations such as Adderall XR, Ritalin LA, Metadate SR, and Concerta.

While the name "Ritalin" has come to represent the whole group of stimulant drugs, Adderall has recently replaced it as the most commonly prescribed stimulant, and a deluge of new pharmaceutical products, including the long-acting agent Concerta, is vying for a large share of the market. Others are continuing to come down the drug-company pipeline. Novartis, the manufacturer of Ritalin, has received FDA approval for a variation on Ritalin named Focalin.

Many parents feel that stimulant drugs are helping their children, and many adults also feel aided by them in controlling ADHD-like behaviors. Chapter 3 of this book will examine the mechanism of action of these drugs and will indicate that the apparent improvement comes at the cost of the overall function of the brain and mind. Other chapters will raise doubts about the efficacy of stimulant drugs for treating "ADHD."

Most children diagnosed with ADHD and treated with stimulants have relatively benign problems. Often they simply daydream in the classroom or dislike school a little more than other children. Or they may be a little more active and energetic than most. Often they are in conflict with one parent but not the other. However, some children diagnosed with ADHD are very angry, out of control, and difficult to be around. When children have these more serious behavioral or emotional problems, stimulant medication is especially likely to worsen their mental condition and behavior. Furthermore, as Chapter 17 will describe, even the most difficult and out-of-control children can be helped by informed adult intervention without resort to drugs.

A Child's Journey Through Psychiatric Diagnoses and Drugs

Since 1968, I have been a psychiatrist in private practice working with both adults and children. Although most of my patients have been adults, I have treated hundreds of children and their families. Over these many years, I have seen dramatic transformations in many aspects of psychiatry, but none as great as recent changes in the treatment of children and youth.

Until recent years, psychiatrists, pediatricians, and other physicians rarely prescribed psychoactive medications for children. As medical doctors, we already had available most of the drugs commonly used to treat children today. We could have prescribed Ritalin or Dexedrine. However, our use of these drugs was restrained by our concern for adverse effects on the growing brain and mind, by awareness of their ineffectiveness, by a broader perspective on the role of families and schools in the lives of children, and by the desire to offer more appropriate psychological, social, and educational services.

Unfortunately, special interests, including drug manufacturers, insurance companies, federal agencies, parent groups, and medical organizations have been pushing physicians to prescribe increasing amounts of medication to children. I have described the activities of these groups in *Talking Back to Ritalin* (rev. ed., 2001a).

The situation has now become truly grim. Not only do doctors routinely prescribe powerful psychoactive substances to children, they increasingly do so in a manner that defies common sense, prudence, and medical science. Hardly a day goes by without several parents or grandparents calling my office to ask my help in salvaging a child who has grossly deteriorated as a result of being prescribed multiple psychiatric drugs, sometimes several at a time.

The Story of Alec

Alec's journey through drug-oriented biological psychiatry will seem uncannily familiar to many parents who have accompanied their children through similar experiences. Stories like this are becoming unfortunately common in modern psychiatry. They are living, painful illustrations of the dangers of the psychiatric diagnosing and drugging of children.

Alec arrived in my office in terrible shape.[1] At the age of eleven, he was physically and psychologically immature. He was skinny, and his ability to control his emotional reactions was minimal. Alec had driven away all his friends, and his older brother never wanted to speak to him again. Even his soccer coach had given up on him, and his school was pushing to transfer him to a facility for the seriously emotionally disturbed.

Alec whined, whimpered, or threw a temper tantrum at the slightest provocation. But it was easy to see the vulnerable, scared kid beneath his manipulative bravado. When he talked about how he "wanted to die" or how "everyone hates me," I saw real despair over his life. When I showed genuine concern for him, he stopped complaining and became eager to hear what I had to say.

By the time he came to see me, Alec had been taking psychiatric drugs for more than five years. His psychiatrist had him on five psychoactive drugs: the long-acting stimulant Concerta, the mood stabilizer Depakote (divalproex), the tranquilizer sedative

Klonopin (clonazepam), the sedating antihypertension agent clonidine, and the adult antipsychotic drug Risperdal (risperidone).

Alec had developed facial twitches and spasms and had lately
been describing how "ghosts" were appearing in his room at
night before he fell asleep. His previous psychiatrist had
explained that Alec was having hallucinations. He warned that
Alec was showing signs of "emerging childhood schizophrenia"
and might need hospitalization for increased medication.

What does a case like this have to do with ADHD?

ADHD was Alec's initial diagnosis at the age of six. At that
time, he was placed on Ritalin. However, he could have been
started on any of the stimulants and the results would probably
have been the same.

I suggested to Alec's parents that we conduct the initial evaluation with the adults and that we then include Alec on a separate
day. I wanted to establish from the start the importance of the
adults getting together to understand the sources and the solutions for Alec's problems. At the start, I wanted to make clear
that Alec's emotional problems did not spring forth, as they had
been previously told, from some abnormality in his brain. I knew
we would find stresses and conflicts in his environment and that
resolving them would set Alec on the right road. While Alec
would have to work on changing his own attitudes and behavior,
his parents and teachers would have to improve their approaches to raising and educating him.

At my suggestion, Alec's parents brought along his maternal
grandmother, who was involved in his everyday care while both
parents worked. Within the first half hour, it became obvious that
the entire family had forgotten a critical fact about Alec's life
story—that Alec had been a normal child at the age of six when
his pediatrician originally started him on Ritalin.

The medicating had begun, as it most often does, with a rec-
ommendation from school for an evaluation. At the start of second grade, Alec's teacher told his parents that he was not paying
attention in class, that he was daydreaming and easily dis-

tractible, and that he sometimes exhibited "ADHD behaviors" such as talking out of turn and leaving his seat without permission. She recommended an evaluation for ADHD and gave them a sheet labeled "Connors Scale," on which she had checked off the specific behaviors that Alec displayed.

The Connors Scale, like the official diagnostic criteria for ADHD, is nothing more than a list of all the behaviors that can require extra attention in a classroom. However, the teacher had attended a workshop on ADHD and had been told the Connors Scale was a valid diagnostic tool for identifying ADHD.

Up to this point, Alec had never been a problem at home. He was a sweet little boy who got along with everyone, even his older brother. However, the pediatrician, after glancing at the Connors Scale, agreed that Alec had ADHD and prescribed Ritalin.

The school and medical records that the parents brought along with them indicated that Alec had "improved" within days after starting on Ritalin. That is, his teacher reported that the little boy was "much nicer to have in class" and that all of the "disruptive behaviors" had disappeared. It seemed like a miracle.

However, within a few months Alec's behavior worsened, and for the first time, he became a little difficult at home. The pediatrician raised the dose of Ritalin, and for a while Alec "improved" again. The pediatrician reassured them that it was just a matter of finding the right dose of stimulant.

Eventually the cycle was repeated several times. With a raise in dose and then with changes in stimulant medication, Alec would temporarily become calmer and easier to be with at home and in school. And then his behavior would get worse than ever before and the medication would be raised or changed again.

In my first session with the adults in the family, it became obvious that the ups and downs on medication kept their hopes alive and obscured the reality that overall the drugs were making him worse.

Within a few weeks after starting Ritalin, his grandmother now remembered, Alec became increasingly "agitated" at night. He became anxious and rebellious, and refused to go to bed. His pediatrician—apparently unaware that stimulants are contraindicated for agitated children—actually increased Alec's Ritalin by adding an afternoon dose. When Alec continued to get more agitated later into the evening, the doctor added the sedative tranquilizer Klonopin to quiet him down and help him sleep.

When Alec's parents forgot on one occasion to bring his medications along on a weekend vacation trip, Alec's behavior deteriorated to a shocking level. He turned into a "monster," requiring physical restraint to prevent him from hurting himself or his family.

Alec's parents made an emergency phone call to the doctor that weekend, but the pediatrician said nothing about Ritalin and Klonopin causing serious withdrawal reactions. He didn't even hint that Alec's deterioration could be an acute withdrawal reaction from Ritalin and Klonopin. Instead, the doctor said Alec should "never stop taking the drugs"—even for the rest of his life. Alec was eight at the time.

Alec's behavior continued to get worse on the medications. Toward the end of third grade, the pediatrician referred the family to a local psychiatrist described as a nationally recognized specialist in treating children with drugs.

The psychiatrist listened to the story and explained, "Your son's bipolar disorder is emerging." The pediatrician's treatment was fine as far as it had gone, he explained, but now an underlying genetic and biological "bipolar disorder" was coming to the surface. He explained that bipolar disorder was another name for manic-depression and that Alec was having mood swings from manic-like irritability to depression. He fully agreed with the pediatrician that Alec would have to take medication for the remainder of his life.

The psychiatrist never mentioned that Ritalin, like any stimulant, can cause extremely out-of-control behavior and that in combination with Klonopin or any tranquilizer, the probability increases for "disinhibition" with a potentially violent loss of emotional control. Instead, the psychiatrist added Depakote to

Alec's regimen, with the intention of controlling his "bipolar disorder."

Alec was now nine and a half years old and going into the fourth grade. When Alec became afraid to go to school and displayed increasing anxiety and agitation, the psychiatrist added an adult antihypertensive agent, clonidine, to the boy's regimen. This brought the total drug regimen to four, including Adderall, Klonopin, Depakote, and clonidine.

The psychiatrist failed to mention that clonidine is not approved for the treatment of any psychiatric disorders. Instead, he told them it was used as a "mood stabilizer." In reality, clonidine is a dangerous drug used to control hypertension in adults that has become a fad treatment for upset children because it tends to heavily sedate them. I have seen children nod off in a session due to clonidine. The psychiatrist also failed to tell them that clonidine and stimulants, in combination, can impair heart function and cause fatal arrhythmias. He did, however, correctly warn them that clonidine could cause a spiking of blood pressure if abruptly stopped.

When Alec's behavior became more violent and explosive on the four drugs, the psychiatrist reaffirmed that Alec had bipolar disorder. During the school year, he changed some of the drug doses and experimented with different kinds of stimulants. Meanwhile, Alec began to talk about killing himself.

In fear and frustration, his parents took Alec for evaluation to a world-famous psychiatrist at the National Institute of Mental Health (NIMH) in Bethesda, Maryland. The new doctor completely approved of "everything" the previous two doctors had done. He did, however, offer a new opinion. Alec's emerging bipolar disorder, he explained, was actually an emerging schizoaffective disorder—a mixture of bipolar disorder and schizophrenia. He added the antipsychotic drug Risperdal to Alec's treatment regimen, for a grand total of five psychiatric drugs, several in adult doses. Alec was now ten and a half years old and weighed less than seventy pounds.

The psychiatrist did not explain that Risperdal is FDA approved only for adults and only for psychoses such as schizophrenia. He also left out something else that by any ethical or medical standard he was especially required to tell the parents, something they would tragically discover on their own.

Three months after starting on Risperdal, Alec began to make odd chewing movements as if struggling with a large gob of gum. His puzzled parents, already frustrated with his behavior, tried to force open his mouth to see what he was chewing. Then they decided he was "making faces" at them, or even worse, at some unseen imaginary person. Soon Alec also began to squint his eyes as if experiencing bursts of glaring light.

When his parents drew Alec's condition to the attention of the NIMH expert, he explained that Alec was showing signs of Tourette's, a disorder of unknown origin that involves a combination of tics and vocalizations. He did not tell them that antipsychotic agents like Risperdal *commonly* cause permanent twitches identical to those that Alec was displaying.

The psychiatrist decided that Alec's increasing reports of "ghosts" and "odd shapes" in his room might be hallucinations caused by his schizophrenic-like illness. He wanted to increase Alec's Risperdal in the hope it would "control" both the tics and the hallucinations.

Indeed, Risperdal—like other antipsychotic agents—can temporarily suppress the very tics and abnormal movements that it causes; but in doing so, it can eventually make them much more disfiguring and even physically disabling.

In my clinical and legal consultations, I have evaluated children whose necks are painfully wrenched out of shape by Risperdal-induced spasms of the neck and shoulders. I've seen children whose eyes periodically roll up in their sockets. I've evaluated another whose breathing is impaired by spasms of the diaphragm.

Children with these drug-induced tics and spasms are among the most tragic cases I have had to evaluate in my work as a psychiatrist. There is no effective treatment for this disorder, and only a few of the children with such obvious tics and spasms have recovered despite months or years off the drugs. Once the disorder has persisted for a few weeks or months, it usually becomes irreversible.

Alec's Grandmother Rescues Him from the Psychiatrist

After Alec started to display these peculiar symptoms, his grandmother began to suspect that the drugs might have something to do with his worsening condition. In libraries and bookstores and on the Web, she began to research the drugs on her own. She came upon one of my books, *Your Drug May Be Your Problem: How and Why to Stop Taking Psychiatric Medications* (1999), coauthored with David Cohen, Ph.D. She learned that Alec's twitches and spasms were tardive dyskinesia, a neurological disorder commonly caused by antipsychotic drugs such as Risperdal, Mellaril, Navane, Prolixin, Thorazine, and Haldol. The FDA requires all antipsychotic drugs (also called neuroleptics) to carry a warning about tardive dyskinesia, including all of the newest antipsychotic drugs like Risperdal, Zyprexa, and Seroquel.

Antipsychotics produce tardive dyskinesia in an astounding 5–8 percent of patients for each year of exposure, for a cumulative rate of 20–32 percent after a mere four years of exposure.[2] With no scientific justification, some doctors got the idea that, unlike other antipsychotics, Risperdal might not produce tardive dyskinesia at such a high rate. This encouraged its widespread prescription to children. I am seeing many cases of Risperdal-induced tardive dyskinesia, and others are being reported in the literature.[3]

After reading my book, Alec's grandmother urged his parents to make an appointment to see me. My practice was full at the time, but when my wife heard the familiar, tragic themes being repeated by Alec's mother on our answering machine, she made it a priority for me to return the call. Alec was now eleven years old and in the fifth grade.

From my initial visit with the parents, it was apparent that psychiatric drugs were destroying Alec. If the process continued, he

would probably end up in adulthood as a chronic mental patient
with disfiguring and even disabling twitches and spasms in his
face and body that would make him look crazy to everyone who
met him. I explained that all of the stimulants can cause or contribute to permanent tics, but less often and usually with less
severity than the antipsychotic drugs. I asked his parents to bring
Alec to my office on an emergency basis that evening.

When I first met Alec, he was displaying the unmistakable signs
of tardive dyskinesia. Although I've been through this many
times before, I was still saddened by what I found. And once
again, I was dismayed that one of my colleagues could have prescribed Risperdal to a child at all and then have gone on to ignore
the devastating results.

The chewing movements and facial tics were already so obvious that Alec's schoolmates were teasing him about them. If
Alec's twitches did not improve or go away, they would gravely
interfere with his social life as he entered his teens. Since they
were affecting his jaw, they could end up impairing his eating and
his teeth. If the drugs weren't stopped, the disorder could progress
to afflict any muscle in his body, from his arms, legs, and torso to
his speech, swallowing, and breathing.[4]

Because Alec had been taking Risperdal for only a few months
and because his parents were willing to stay in close touch with
me, I planned a rapid one-week taper. Within a week, his parents
already felt that he seemed "much more like our Alec." However, his tics and spasms temporarily worsened, as they often do
during the withdrawal period after the drugs are reduced in
dosage or stopped.

Working with Alec

Alec was a spirited, courageous child struggling with all his might
to contend with the confusion in his life and the toxins in his
brain. I could easily find the sweet and gentle boy who had
thrived before the advent of psychiatric drugs in his life.

I explained to Alec that his story indicated that he didn't have any kind of psychiatric disorder and that most of his disturbed behavior came from a combination of the drugs and his parents' difficulties in learning to discipline him. I further explained that it would require a great deal of work on his part to learn to control his behavior.

Alec was reassured when I reminded him that before the drugs, he had no problem controlling his behavior as well as any other kid. He responded with surprising eagerness to my explanations about how hard he would have to work to get his behavior back under control.

Then Alec demanded, "What about them?" and made a vigorous gesture in his parents' direction. I explained that he should refer to his parents in a more respectful manner. He could tell I was serious about this, and to his parents' surprise, he agreed to this as well. I went on to tell him that when he did ask a question respectfully, I would always try to answer him. In that spirit, I explained that his parents and grandmother would indeed have their own work to do. They would have to develop a more consistent, rational plan of discipline for him and would have to find more time to spend with him.

"It's clear your parents and your grandmother love you," I explained, "but they've been misled by doctors into thinking that you can't control your behavior and that they can't help you get control over yourself. This has been very harmful to the whole family. We'll be able to fix this situation quickly if everyone can get together on a plan for more self-restraint and more respect in the family."

"If you say so, Doc," Alec said, and then, laughing at his own disrespectful tone of voice and demonstrating his capacity for self-control, he added more respectfully, "Dr. Breggin." I laughed, too. I liked this spirited child.

After rapidly stopping Alec's Risperdal on an emergency basis, I continued to remove Alec from his other drugs over the next few months. His parents were deeply grateful to see their son returning to them. During this time, I worked with the entire family and on occasion with Alec's teachers and principal on how to handle his sometimes difficult behavior.

When alone with Alec on occasion, I emphasized that changing his behavior was not "giving in" to adults as he feared. I explained how it was actually in his own self-interest to gain more self-discipline and responsibility. Children are much more able to respond to rational discussion than most health-care professionals seem to realize. They want to know why and how they should change their behavior. Unfortunately, not one of Alec's previous physicians had talked with him about his inherent capacity to control his conduct, why he should want to do so, and how he could go about it.

Alec grew several inches in the first year under my care and filled out as well. His posture changed from an angry slouch to a proud erect carriage, and his facial expression transformed from somber defiance into reflection of a full range of normal and often high-spirited emotions.

Alec's grades went from flunking across the board to mostly C's and then to a mixture of A's and B's. He was once again becoming the bright child he had been before he started taking psychiatric drugs.

After Alec was free of psychiatric drugs for several months, he became one of the few fortunate children whose tardive dyskinesia almost completely resolved. A careful examination still discloses some abnormal movements of his tongue and jaw, especially if he is stressed or fatigued, but if noticed by anyone they are likely to seem like nervous habits. Alec probably recovered so well because his grandmother became suspicious as soon as the tics developed and we were able to stop the drugs before he had taken them for months or years.

Alec and his parents stopped coming regularly for treatment after about two years, but I continue to hear from Alec occasionally. He likes to call to say hello once in a while. He's doing well in regular classes in public high school, presents no serious behavior problems in the classroom or home, and is even getting along better with his older brother. He is looking forward to going to college. Now that he no longer thinks of himself as mentally ill and now that his brain is free of toxins, I am sure he will continue to blossom.

Alec should never have been put on psychiatric drugs. His inattention and restlessness in the classroom in the second grade could have been handled with more patience, attention to his needs, and better teaching methods. At that time, he didn't have problems at home, but if he had been a "difficult child," that too could have been handled with improved parenting. There was no reason whatsoever to expose this child to any psychoactive substances, let alone a several-year regimen of multiple psychiatric drugs. In my experience, children do not need psychoactive agents. They need improved adult attention to their basic needs for discipline, love, and inspired teaching.

Is Alec's story unusual? No, his story is being repeated with hundreds of thousands and perhaps millions of children throughout America. Almost all of these children have conflicts with adults that could be handled by improved, individualized approaches to teaching and parenting. Instead, a doctor starts them on a stimulant drug such as Ritalin, Concerta, or Adderall; the drugs cause new problems, and the child ends up on multiple psychoactive substances. In this way, the stimulants can become the gateway to a lifetime on multiple psychiatric drugs. Meanwhile, doctors who advocate drugs will often ignore and even openly deny that the drugs could be causing any of the problems, even after the child begins to have persisting tics and spasms induced by stimulants like Ritalin and Adderall, or more likely by antipsychotic drugs like Risperdal.

The following chapters will look at the scientific evidence confirming the wide variety of psychiatric and physical disorders that can be caused by the stimulant drugs.

3

Of Cages and Creativity—
How Stimulants Work

If you are considering the use of stimulant drugs for yourself or your children, you probably want answers to the following questions:

Do stimulants really help children?
How do they work?
Are they dangerous?

In response to these questions, too many doctors tell parents and patients that stimulants work well and have few if any serious risks. They may also explain that the drugs work by "correcting biochemical imbalances" or "improving focus and attention."

This chapter addresses the question "How do the stimulants work?" It reveals the manner in which stimulant drugs actually change the behavior of children and adults. The facts are both surprising and shocking.

How Can a Stimulant Help "Overstimulated" Children?

People are often puzzled by the use of a "stimulant" drug to treat children who seem in many ways to be "overstimulated." They wonder, "How can a stimulant help a child who already seems 'hyper' and 'out of control'?"

Some professionals used to believe that stimulants work differently in children than in adults, but informed experts have known for decades that this is not the case. There is nothing unique about the impact of stimulants on children other than the tendency to cause more adverse or harmful effects in the young brain.

Stimulants do in fact overstimulate many children. There is a continuum of stimulation, with insomnia, irritability, and tension (feeling "hyper") at the lower level of intensity. As the dose increases, so do the likelihood and intensity of overstimulation, with symptoms of worsening insomnia, irritability, tension, anxiety, and agitation. At the extreme end of the continuum of stimulation, the drugs can cause an out-of-control "high" in the form of manic reactions, psychotic symptoms, and violence. The stimulant effects can cause cardiac problems, hypertension, and convulsions. Based on the FDA-approved labels, I have summarized these symptoms of stimulant toxicity in the next chapter (see Table 4.1).

This stimulation is not the desired or hoped-for therapeutic effect. Stimulation is an adverse effect that actually worsens the child's condition.

Because the drug is stimulating, the official Ritalin label in the 2001 *Physicians' Desk Reference* warns: "Marked anxiety, tension, and agitation are contraindications to Ritalin, since the drug may aggravate these symptoms." Similarly, the Adderall label warns that it should not be given to people in "agitated states." These remarkable statements are contained in the section entitled "Contraindications." Ritalin is actually contraindicated—that is, it's not supposed to be given—for children with "marked anxiety, tension, and agitation." Yet doctors often mistakenly give Ritalin, Adderall, and other stimulants to children who suffer from these problems.

The stimulating effects of Ritalin are further confirmed on its label by the observation, "Nervousness and insomnia are the most common adverse reactions . . . " Similarly, the Adderall label describes "overstimulation," "restlessness," "insomnia," and "euphoria" as adverse reactions. The Ritalin label warns, "Toxic psychosis has been reported." The Adderall label further notes the existence of drug-induced "psychotic episodes at recommended doses (rare)."

Notice that the psychotic episodes can occur at "recommended" doses, that is, within the accepted range of routine treatment. In the section on overdose, the Dexedrine and Adderall labels mention that the whole range of "toxic" symptoms can occasionally occur at low doses. In fact, all the toxic stimulant symptoms including cardiac arrhythmias, agitation, and hallucinations can occur at routine doses (see Chapter 5). The stimulating effects of drugs such as Ritalin, Adderall, and Focalin become more frequent and blatantly obvious when there is an accidental or intentional overdose, but they can occur even at small doses.

Many physicians seem to miss the reality that stimulants often overstimulate children, making them more nervous, tense, anxious, and agitated, and therefore more uncontrollable and ADHD-like in their behavior. When the child's behavior worsens, instead of stopping the drug altogether, these misinformed doctors will often increase the dosage or add another drug, ultimately worsening the child's condition.

How Stimulants "Work"

When I was a child, I was always delighted to hear the Good Humor ice-cream truck when it came creeping down the street amid its charming jingle of bells. I never saw one of those trucks go fast and learned that they had governors on their engines—devices that prevented the truck from speeding. Stifling the truck's natural horsepower helped protect neighborhood children from potentially reckless ice-cream-truck drivers.

All stimulants—including Ritalin, Adderall, Focalin, and Concerta—work by putting a governor on the child's brain, literally suppressing the brain's ability to generate spontaneous mental life and behavior. We know this from many animal studies spanning several decades. These same effects are also seen in normal as well as distressed children and adults.

Suppressing Caged Rats

Humans share the same basic brain structure as smaller mammals. The same functional components with the same neurotransmitter (chemical messenger) systems exist in humans and animals alike. Therefore, animal studies can tell us a great deal about a drug's basic effects on behavior. In fact, efforts to find new psychiatric drugs always involve initial testing on animals.

For example, anesthetics that create unconsciousness in preparation for surgery, analgesics that reduce pain, and sedatives that calm anxiety and produce sleep cause similar observable effects in humans and animals alike.

Stimulants have similar effects on humans as they do on rats and chimpanzees. I have known people who made pets out of rats, which can be rather endearing animals. They are playful, inquisitive, and active. Your pet rat delights in climbing all over you, sniffing you wherever possible, and exploring every inch of its available environment.

All animals including human beings are motivated to explore their world and to learn everything they can about it. Survival depends upon our insatiable curiosity about our environment. This characteristic is most obvious in the young of all species, who, often to the consternation of their parents, delight in endless play and dangerous explorations. Indeed, many adults retain these childhood qualities and desire a considerable portion of exploration, play, and socialization in their daily lives.

From rats to chimpanzees and humans, we also share a dislike of confinement. Put any creature in a cage or a box, and escape becomes its first priority.

Making Good Caged Animals

What happens if rats or chimpanzees are given clinical doses of stimulant drugs such as Ritalin, Focalin, Concerta, or Adderall?

Dozens of scientific studies have given us a very consistent and comprehensive answer.[1]

The stimulant drug transforms them from active, inquisitive animals into compulsive, dull creatures. Pick any self-generated behavior and it is likely to be crushed, including exploration, inquisitiveness, socialization, and escape behavior. Play, that most important method of learning, is typically reduced to zero.

How do the drugs accomplish this? Stimulants disrupt the connections in the highest developmental regions of the brain, including the frontal lobes, which are the seat of the most advanced behaviors of any species. When these areas are damaged in animals or humans, the most complex and subtle functions are flattened or destroyed. It's a kind of chemical lobotomy.

Animals and children given stimulants don't become entirely inactive. Instead, they become narrowly focused and compulsive in their behavior. For example, the animal will stop trying to escape its cage and instead pace endlessly back and forth in a small corner. Or the animal will stop looking with interest outside the cage and instead stare hypnotically at small objects on the ground. Some animals will develop obsessive-compulsive behaviors, such as chewing on their paws, picking at their skin, or gnawing on the bars of the cage. These repetitive behaviors are called "perseveration" or "stereotypy." By definition they are dysfunctional, meaningless behaviors caused by brain dysfunction.

Our nearest animal cousins, chimpanzees, like to socialize in ways quite similar to people. They kiss and hug, and especially like to groom each other. On clinical doses of stimulants, chimps stop socializing and stop mutual grooming. Instead, they will sit by themselves and groom their own bodies in a narrowly focused fashion, picking at one or two areas, sometimes until their skin becomes raw. While their behaviors will vary, their reactions to clinical doses of stimulants have this quality of reduced spontaneity, social isolation, and repeated meaningless behaviors. For example, a series of recent studies of small doses of stimulants found the following effects: compulsive picking at the skin, repetitive fiddling with things, static posturing, aimless pacing, inappropriate responses that had no relationship to any stimulus, staring off into space, social withdrawal, and increased submissiveness.[2] All of these behaviors, including increased submissiveness, are also found in human children after they have been given stimulants.

To the casual observer, the crushing of spontaneity makes the animals seem "happier" in their cages and more accepting of their captivity. At least, they show fewer or less intense signs of their distress at being confined. They don't struggle to get out of the cage; they don't look mournfully at their neighbors who are caged beyond their reach. But they aren't happier; they are duller. Their natural enthusiasm for life has been snuffed out.

Compared to advocates of stimulant drugs, the animal researchers are much more aware of the actual impact of the drugs. For example, animal researchers will describe stimulant-induced obsessive behaviors as "meaningless" or "lacking in spontaneity." Meanwhile, drug advocates will describe the same behavior in children as an improvement because the child is now willing to do rote school activities and to sit still in class without talking to his or her neighbors.

Professional Ignorance About the Facts

Do the advocates of stimulants know about these animal behavior studies? Most of them do not. Even those who should know seem not to know or care.

After I was asked by the director's office of the National Institutes of Health (NIH) to be the scientific presenter on adverse drug effects in children at the Consensus Development Conference on the Diagnosis and Treatment of Attention Deficit Hyperactivity Disorder, I talked about my presentation to the organizer of the conference, psychiatrist Peter Jensen. At the time, Jensen was on the staff of the National Institute of Mental Health. He is now at Columbia University. Jensen is one of the world's most staunch and presumably informed advocates of stimulant drugs for children. I explained to him that in addition to discussing adverse drug effects during my scientific presentation to the consensus conference, I also wanted to discuss animal research showing how the drugs have "therapeutic" effects on behavior. Jensen was surprised that any such literature existed. When I told him there were innumerable scientific studies and described them to him, he acted completely surprised.

Observing Children in the Classroom

The effectiveness of stimulant drugs is often "proven" by asking teachers to rate the behavior of children in a classroom setting. The teachers will be given checklists to fill out for the children containing items that are used in the official diagnostic manual to determine if a child has ADHD. This *Diagnostic and Statistical Manual of Mental Disorders, IV* is published by the American Psychiatric Association (1994). It contains items such as "often fidgets with hands or feet or squirms in seat," "often leaves seat in classroom," "often blurts out answers," "has difficulty awaiting turn," and "often does not seem to listen."

Teachers and parents almost always report a reduction of these kinds of behaviors in children given stimulants.[3] The teachers and parents have not been told that this involves a suppression of spontaneous behavior with enforced submissiveness and so they fail to recognize that the drugs are suppressing or dulling the children.

Teachers are especially likely to find that the children are "improved" because they are asked to rate behaviors such as "blurts out answers" or "leaves seat" that are especially reduced when overall spontaneity is crushed. The reduction in spontaneous behavior, as well as the enforced submissiveness, makes the children less talkative, less likely to leave their seats, and less likely to socialize with their neighbors. These reductions in overall spontaneous behavior make it easier for teachers to run their classrooms without having to pay attention to the individual child.

Exactly as in the animal studies, stimulants also make children more compulsive. For the chimpanzees, this means sitting by themselves while they groom one small spot on the arm or play endlessly with a pebble. For our children, this drug-enforced compulsivity makes them focus on previously unendurable boring tasks such as copying from the board or writing something down ten times. These children often become so compulsive that they bear down too hard on the paper as they write or persist at the task even when asked to stop. Studies describe them as abnormally overfocused. However, teachers and parents are likely to mistake such behavior for a genuine "buckling down" on schoolwork and homework.

Table 3.1 is entitled "Harmful Stimulant Drug Reactions Commonly Misidentified as 'Therapeutic' or 'Beneficial.'"[4] When children are given Ritalin, Adderall, and other stimulant drugs, they frequently develop these kinds of reactions. Unfortunately, researchers, doctors, teachers, and parents routinely misinterpret these toxic effects as improvements in the children.

Do the children learn better? Are their scholastic abilities improved? Of course not. Drug-induced impairments cannot make a child wiser, more thoughtful, or better informed. They can only make children sit down, shut up, and do what they are told. As we shall see, there is no evidence that stimulant drugs actually improve academic performance. But they do sometimes lead to improved grades because many teachers will reward more submissive, unobtrusive behavior with better grades.

Some of the staunchest advocates of stimulants for children have in effect admitted that the drugs work by enforcing blind obedience. Russell Barkley, one of the most widely published Ritalin/ADHD advocates, uses the term "compliance" to describe this improved behavior. Stimulant drugs do indeed tend to make children more compliant, that is, more manageable and obedient. They do so at the expense of their imaginations, their creativity, their capacity to generate activity, and their overall enthusiasm for life.

TABLE 3.1 Harmful Stimulant Drug Reactions Commonly Misidentified as "Therapeutic" or "Beneficial," Selected from 20 Controlled Clinical Trials Involving Children Diagnosed with ADHD

Obsessive Compulsive Effects	Social Withdrawal Effects	Behaviorally Suppressive Effects
Compulsive persistence at meaningless activities (called stereotypical or perseverative behavior)	Social withdrawal and isolation	Compliant in structured environments; socially inhibited, passive, and submissive
	General dampened social behavior	Somber, subdued, apathetic, lethargic, dopey, dazed, and tired
Increased obsessive-compulsive behavior (e.g., repeating chores endlessly and ineffectively)	Reduced communication and socialization	Bland, emotionally flat, humorless, not smiling, depressed, and sad with frequent crying
Mental rigidity (called cognitive perseveration)	Decreased responsiveness to parents and other children	Lacking in initiative, spontaneity, curiosity, surprise, or pleasure
Inflexible thinking	Increased solitary play and diminished overall play	
Overly narrow or excessive focusing		

Modified from Breggin (1999b, 1999c), reprinted by permission of Springer Publishing Co. References to the 20 clinical trials provided in Breggin (1999b, 1999c).

However, as the brain resists the drug's effect, the child can become even more distressed and unmanageable. Alec's story in Chapter 2 illustrates this kind of worsening of behavior that increases over time without doctors or parents attributing it to the medication itself. Before medication, improved teaching and parenting could have genuinely helped the child. But now the child suffers from drug-induced impairments that interfere with taking responsibility and learning self-control. In my clinical experience, many children who take these drugs for several years remain more immature and less able to manage on their own. The same outcome can be observed with illicit drug abuse.

Drug-Impaired Attention

Attention is among the highest human capacities. When I'm writing a book, for example, I have to be able to block out unwanted stimulation and focus on the tasks ahead. An athlete must have the ability to focus on the immediate challenge, just as anyone facing a difficult task must learn to focus on the essentials. This is also apparent in grade school, where children must learn to set priorities in regard to homework and then select and focus on specific activities. Attention of this kind requires personal motivation, rational choice making, and persistent acts of will power. Teachers and parents can play a positive role by guiding the child's spontaneous interests in rewarding directions.

The kind of "attention" produced by stimulant drugs does not involve the making of rational choices or acts of will. It is an enforced obsessive-compulsive attention to rote activities.[5] Personal choice plays little or no role. The child does not feel personally motivated and does not independently, rationally choose to pay attention. Instead, the child's natural desire to pay attention to other things, such as playing on the computer or socializing with friends, is diminished or even crushed by a corresponding loss of brain function. The child becomes more obedient without learning to be self-motivated, to make rational choices, and to exert will power.

Studies described in Chapter 4 will confirm that children on stimulants commonly become lethargic, apathetic, or otherwise lacking in spontaneity. They smile, joke, and play with less intensity and frequency. Sometimes the suppression is so extreme that the children are diagnosed as depressed or described as zombie-like.

Relief for Parents and Teachers

Parents and teachers who feel overwhelmed by the effort required to control their classrooms or homes are likely to view a reduction in spontaneous behavior as an improvement in their children or students. If the parent or teacher hasn't been informed about what's really happening, it may seem like a miracle cure when a rambunctious or difficult child becomes more socially withdrawn, less spontaneous, more compliant, and more willing to put up with really boring activities.

Often the drug effect is so subtle as to be hardly discernible. The child does not appear grossly less spontaneous or more isolated. The child is simply easier to be around. For many overtaxed parents and teachers, this can feel like a blessing.

Am I saying that these drugs never really help children? Yes, I am. While children may become more docile and easier to manage and may sometimes do more of their homework assignments or chores, their more docile or seemingly cooperative behavior is the result of drug-induced impairments in spontaneity and concentration. They are not learning to be more self-disciplined or genuinely cooperative; the drugs are chronically impairing their brains.

Many parents notice that the drugs have robbed them of their children. They tell me that the drugs caused their children to lose their "luster" or "spark." Their personalities were "changed" in negative ways. In more extreme reactions, the children seemed to "lose their soul" and become "robotic."

"Correcting Biochemical Imbalances"

Recently I gave a lecture to students and professionals at a medical center. Initially, some of them were surprised when I explained that all psychoactive drugs disrupt normal brain function. They, too, had been misled by drug-company propaganda to believe that psychiatric drugs correct biochemical imbalances. However, several were immediately able to see the truth once I reminded them about the facts.

Research on psychoactive drugs almost always begins with animal studies. As a first step, a series of animal brains will be examined to measure the normal activity of a specific function, such as the rate of firing of a particular type of brain cell (neuron). Tiny electrodes may be inserted into the brains to measure the activity of the cells. Or the animal brain may be removed in order to determine the normal amount of a specific chemical in the region.

Next, a new series of animals will be given the stimulant drug, such as Ritalin or Adderall. Then their brains will be examined to determine how the drug changes these normal functions. For example, the brain cells may begin to fire more rapidly than normal for a while and then, later on, more slowly than normal. Or the specific chemical messenger may increase above normal in amount for a while and then decrease below normal later on.

The pharmacological action of any psychoactive drug is demonstrated by how it disrupts the normal function of an animal's brain. That disruption is the basis of the psychoactive effect. The researchers, the drug company, the FDA, and everyone else involved in the field will then assume that the drug disrupts human brain function in exactly the same fashion. When textbooks or reviews discuss the drug's "mode of action," they will simply describe what has been learned from research on how the drug interferes with the functioning of the normal animal brain.

However, when the drug company and its experts get ready to present this information to the medical profession and the public, they will perform remarkable verbal sleights of hand. The known fact that the drug disrupts normal brain function will be ignored and instead the drug will be falsely promoted as correcting bio-chemical imbalances. The claim about correcting biochemical imbalances is a deliberate deception to make the drugs look positive. Similarly, the known fact that the drug suppresses behavior will be ignored, and in the case of the stimulants, nothing at all will be said about it. How the drug actually works will remain shrouded in mystery.

The Brain Scan Scam

In an attempt to justify the drugging of children, various pro-drug researchers have tried to show that children diagnosed with ADHD have different brains than ordinary or normal children. On the face of it, this makes no sense, since the diagnosis of ADHD, as based on the American Psychiatric Association's *Diagnostic and Statistical Manual of Mental Disorders, IV,* is nothing but a catchall list of every kind of behavior that can disrupt a classroom. How can that have a physiological basis? Instead, the behaviors described as ADHD can be caused by anything from boring teachers and overcrowded classrooms to poorly taught discipline in the home. Often, parents and teachers have unreasonable expectations for normal children.

So how do drug advocates manage to come up with studies that demonstrate abnormalities in the brain scans of children diagnosed with ADHD? First of all, they don't really come up with any consistent findings. Their studies typically contradict each other. More important, almost all the studies that find brain abnormalities have been conducted on children who have been exposed to multiple psychiatric drugs for months or years prior to the brain scans (see Chapter 5). We know that all psychoactive drugs can harm the brain, but the pro-drug researchers never take this into account.

In conclusion, the seemingly beneficial effects of stimulants are in fact the result of harmful drug effects on the brain and mind. Stimulants work by impairing normal brain function. The child becomes less spontaneously active, more submissive, and more willing to focus on boring, rote tasks. For parents and teachers who feel at a loss in dealing with these children, these results can seem miraculous. These parents and teachers need to know that the children are being biochemically impaired and injured by the drugs and that, in the long run, the drugs will do much more harm than good.

How Stimulants Cause Psychiatric Disorders

Stimulants are powerful psychoactive substances that impact the brain and mind. We have already seen that their primary or therapeutic impact involves flattening all spontaneous behavior, enforcing submissiveness, and causing obsessive focus on rote activities. Therefore, it should be no surprise that they can cause a variety of other mental abnormalities.

In reviewing adverse drug reaction reports made to the FDA concerning Ritalin, I found hundreds of cases of Ritalin-induced psychiatric reactions.[1] Children taking Ritalin were most commonly reported to develop—in the following order—agitation, hostility, depression and psychotic depression, abnormal thinking, hallucinations, psychosis, and emotional instability (called "lability"). There were many reports of overdose, intentional overdose, and suicide attempts, confirming the risk of depression and potential suicide.

Causing Toxic Stimulation

Chapter 3 described the continuum of stimulant effects that can occur at any dose but that usually increase in frequency and severity with increasing doses. Of great importance, some individuals will have very severe stimulant reactions at low doses. The stimulant effects that manifest as psychiatric problems include insomnia, irritability, anxiety, agitation, aggression, confusion or delirium, and psychosis. Stimulants often worsen ADHD-like symptoms such as inattention and difficulty focusing and can cause loss of impulse control and aggression.

The stimulants also cause a variety of physical disorders, including the potential for hypertension, hypotension, cardiac arrhythmias, and even shock with circulatory collapse. They can also cause convulsions.

I have taken several approaches to summarizing the overall adverse effects of stimulants. Table 3.1 (in Chapter 3) uses data from twenty clinical trials to describe adverse psychiatric effects such as apathy, depression, and overfocusing that are commonly mistaken for improvements in children's behavior.

Table 4.1, "Toxic Reactions to Stimulants: Usually in Overdose and Occasionally at Low Doses," is drawn entirely from the "Overdose" sections of the official FDA-approved labels for Ritalin, Dexedrine, Adderall, and Adderall XR. Almost any adverse reaction that occurs in overdose can also occur at lower doses.

For an overview of stimulant effects taken from a broader variety of medical sources other than the drug labels, see Table 4.2, "Overview of Harmful Reactions to Stimulant Drugs: Ritalin, Dexedrine, Adderall, Concerta, and Metadate."

Tables 3.1, 4.1, and 4.2 cover most of the adverse effects of stimulants that are likely to show up in routine clinical use. They are compiled from standard or mainstream sources that tend to approve or advocate the use of stimulant drugs. There is a great tendency in the medical literature to minimize adverse drug effects in order to support or promote the use of medications in general. Therefore, the individual sources are not as comprehensive as the data that I have compiled in this book from all of the sources. *In addition, few if any sources fully address the brain damage and dysfunction produced by these drugs, including*

TABLE 4.1   Toxic Reactions to Stimulants: Usually in Overdose and Occasionally at Low Doses

Agitation	Elevated heart rate
Tremors	Palpitations
Increased neurologic reflexes	Cardiac arrhythmias
Muscle twitching	Hypertension
Convulsions	Enlarged pupils
Coma	Dry mouth, nose, and eyes
Euphoria	Increased respiration[a]
Confusion	Nausea, vomiting, diarrhea,
Hallucinations	and cramps[a]
Delirium	Muscle breakdown[a]
Sweating	Hypotension, shock, and
Flushing	circulatory collapse[a]
Headache	Panic states[a]
High fever	Assaultiveness[a]

[a]Indicates the item was taken from the FDA-approved overdose section of the labels for Dexedrine, Adderall, and Adderall XR, but not Ritalin. The remainder was taken from the Ritalin label with some overlap. The Dexedrine and Adderall labels both state that "individual patient response to amphetamines varies widely" and "toxic symptoms occasionally occur as an idiosyncrasy at doses as low as 2 mg." The Adderall XR label also states that patient responses "vary widely" and "toxic symptoms" may occur "at low doses." *Most of the symptoms can occur with any of the stimulants at routine clinical doses.*

strong evidence for stimulant-induced brain shrinkage, cell death, and persistent biochemical changes. These will be described in Chapter 5 (see Table 5.1).

When Doctors Told the Truth

In 1992, a team of experts selected by the U.S. Department of Education was asked to examine the entire body of stimulant literature and to publish a review concerning the effects of the drugs.[2] The experts made sobering observations on the harmful effects of stimulants on mental processes. The team found that "cognitive toxicity may occur at commonly prescribed clinical doses of stimulant medication." "Cognitive toxicity" means a deterioration of mental functions such as thinking, learning,

TABLE 4.2 Overview of Harmful Reactions to Stimulant Drugs: Ritalin, Dexedrine, Adderall, Concerta, and Metadate

Brain and Mind Function
Obsessive-compulsive behavior
Zombie-like (robotic) behavior with loss of emotional spontaneity
Drowsiness, "dopey," reduced alertness
Abnormal movements, tics, Tourette's
Nervous habits (picking at skin, pulling hair)
Convulsions
Headache
Stroke
Mania, psychosis
Visual and tactile hallucinations
Agitation, anxiety, nervousness
Insomnia
Irritability, hostility, aggression
Depression, suicide, easy crying, social withdrawal
Confusion, mental impairments (decreased cognition and learning)
Stimulant addiction and abuse

Gastrointestinal Function
Anorexia
Nausea, vomiting, bad taste
Stomachache
Cramps
Dry mouth
Constipation, diarrhea
Liver dysfunction

Withdrawal and Rebound Reactions
Insomnia
Excessive sleep
Evening crash
Depression
Rebound worsening of ADHD-like symptoms
Overactivity and irritability

Endocrine and Metabolic Function
Pituitary dysfunction, including growth hormone and prolactin disruption
Weight loss
Growth suppression
Disturbed sexual function

Cardiovascular Function
Hypertension
Abnormal heartbeat
Heart disease
Cardiac arrest

Other Functions
Blurred vision
Hair loss
Dizziness
Hypersensitivity reaction with rash

Modified from Breggin (1999a, 1999c) by permission of Springer Publishing Company. Sources include Arnold and Jensen (1995, Table 38-5, pp. 2306–2307; Table 38-7; and p. 2307), Drug Enforcement Administration (1995b, p. 23), Dulcan (1994, Table 35-6, p. 1217), Maxmen and Ward (1995, pp. 365–366), and Food and Drug Administration (1997, March).

attention, and memory. They also warned about "zombie-like" behavior. Citing many scientific sources, the researchers made the following observations:

> In some disruptive children, drug-induced compliant behavior may be accompanied by isolated, withdrawn, and overfocused behavior. Some medicated children may seem "zombie-like" and high doses which make ADHD children more "somber," "quiet," and "still" may produce social isolation by increasing "time spent alone" and decreasing "time spent in positive interaction" on the playground.

They emphasized the danger of "overfocusing of attention which may impair rather than improve learning if taken to an extreme."

According to this report sponsored by the Department of Education, cognitive toxicity from Ritalin is common—occurring in "40% or more of the typically treated cases." As two other experienced researchers confirmed, the cognitive toxicity manifests itself "in the realm of complex, higher-order cognitive functions such as flexible problem-solving and divergent thinking."[3] In other words, many children are being forced to overfocus at the expense of their overall ability to think and learn.

Psychiatric Drugs: A Major Cause of Psychiatric Disability

In 1984, Fialkov and Hasley at the Western Psychiatric Institute and Clinic in Pittsburgh found that 66 percent of psychiatrically hospitalized children had been taking multiple psychiatric drugs prior to the worsening of their condition. They warned "that inappropriate and injudicious use of psychotropic medications may be associated with unanticipated adverse behavioral effects, which can result in deterioration of a child's functioning to the point of necessitating psychiatric hospitalization."

That was many years ago; the situation is much worse now in regard to prescribing multiple medications to children.

Stimulants Commonly Cause Mental Disorders

Stimulants commonly cause a variety of serious emotional disturbances. I am not alone in drawing this conclusion. A handbook frequently used by physicians lists the following rates of adverse mental effects caused by stimulants:[4]

TABLE 4.3   Rates of Adverse Mental Effects Reported in Stimulant Clinical Trials

Adverse Stimulant Effect	Amphetamines (Dexedrine, Adderall)	Methylphenidate (Ritalin, Concerta, Metadate ER)
Drowsiness, less alert	5.5%	5.7%
Confused, "dopey"	10.3% (8–12%)	3.9% (2–10%)
Depression	39%	8.7%
Agitation, restlessness	More than 10%	6.7% (3.3% to more than 10%)
Irritability, stimulation	25% (17–29%)	17.3% (11–19%)

The data are from Maxmen and Ward (1995, p. 366). The numbers are percentages of patients reported in studies to suffer from the adverse effects. Numbers in parentheses represent the range reported in studies.

The rates in this chart are drawn from clinical studies. Not many parents would expose their children to these drugs if they were aware of the frequency with which the drugs can impair a child's mental life.

The studies are usually conducted by advocates for drugs and tend to minimize adverse drug reactions. Therefore, most of the rates are actually higher than reported in the chart. While the rates for these adverse effects vary widely from study to study, the main point is inescapable: Stimulants frequently harm the brain and mind.

As a part of my scientific presentation at the NIH Consensus Development Conference on the Diagnosis and Treatment of Attention Deficit Hyperactivity Disorder in 1998, I reviewed eight representative controlled clinical trials to estimate the frequency of adverse effects. All of the studies were conducted by advocates of stimulants and aimed at proving that the drugs are safe and effective. I have reviewed them in the scientific literature[5] and in *Talking Back to Ritalin* (rev. ed., 2001a). Based on these studies, I estimate that the reported rate of serious adverse reactions in children was as high as 10–20 percent or more.[6] The real rate in clinical practice would be even higher.

In reviewing Table 4.3, it is important to realize that symptoms such as "irritability," "agitation," and "confused" are related to each other. They reflect gross underlying brain dysfunctions that then become manifested in varying ways. When brain function is disrupted in such a global or generalized way, almost any mental abnormality or mixture of abnormalities can result.

Causing Depression and Apathy

My clinical experience confirms the data in Table 4.3: Children taking stimulants frequently become very depressed and even suicidal. Their doctors often fail to recognize the source of the depression. Instead of stopping the stimulant medication, they add an antidepressant, causing even greater emotional disturbances in the child.

How common is stimulant-induced depression? Very common!

The rate of 39 percent for amphetamine-induced depression cited in Table 4.3 may seem surprisingly high. However, it is consistent with another estimate from the U.S. Drug Enforcement Administration (1995b) that more than 20 percent of children on stimulants will become depressed.

A 1997 study published in *Pediatrics* confirms high rates of stimulant-induced depression in 125 children ages five to fifteen treated for ADHD who were given relatively small doses of Ritalin or Dexedrine.[7] Two children on Ritalin and two on Dexedrine developed severe enough adverse effects to be terminated from the study. One eight-year-old became "over-focused, extra sensitive, and increasingly anxious," and a five-year-old became "extremely aggressive and tearful." Signs of drug-induced depression were very common, with statistically significant increases in trouble sleeping, poor appetite, headaches, nightmares, biting fingernails, and being "unusually unhappy."

When parents tell physicians that they have heard about the controversy surrounding Ritalin, some doctors will, in a misleading fashion, explain that they have alternative drugs, such as Adderall and Dexedrine. However, these amphetamines are no safer than Ritalin. In the 1997 study, side effects from amphetamine (Dexedrine) were higher than those from Ritalin for "trouble sleeping, irritability, prone to crying, anxiousness, sadness/ unhappiness, and nightmares."

A 1994 study of 69 children ages two to thirteen given Ritalin also confirmed the frequency of adverse reactions and depression.[8] Six of the children discontinued the study, and 13 (8.8 percent) became "significantly worse" on the drug. A total of 18 percent suffered from "lethargy." Children diagnosed with "lethargy" were actually showing signs of depression. They were "variously described by raters as tired, withdrawn, listless, depressed, dopey, dazed, subdued, and inactive."

Causing Psychosis

The "Warnings" section of the 2002 Ritalin label states: "Clinical experience suggests that in psychotic children, administration of Ritalin may exacerbate symptoms of behavior disturbance and thought disorder." The 2002 Adderall XR label, found on the Shire US Inc. web site,[9] states: "Clinical experience suggests that, in psychotic patients, administration of amphetamine may exacerbate symptoms of behavioral disturbance and thought disorder." In other words, Adderall XR, like any amphetamine, can worsen behavioral problems and psychosis. Under "Adverse Reactions," the labels for both drugs give further recognition to the danger of making children and adults psychotic. The Ritalin label refers succinctly to this fact: "Toxic psychosis has been reported." The Adderall XR label notes "psychotic episodes at recommended doses." Thus, stimulants can not only exacerbate behavioral disturbances and psychosis, they can flat out cause them "at recommended doses."

Too many doctors do not know that stimulants commonly make children "crazy." In my earlier writings, my own estimate of 1 percent for stimulant-induced psychosis was too low. It was based on observations in the literature that can now be updated on the basis of continuing research.

An October 1999 review examined psychiatric clinic charts of ninety-eight children spanning five years. The children were diagnosed with ADHD and treated with stimulants. They were compared to similar children diagnosed with ADHD who were not treated with stimulants. Nine percent of the drug-treated children developed psychotic symptoms during treatment, while none of the drug-free children developed these problems.[10] Seven of the children who became disturbed were taking Ritalin, and two were taking the non-amphetamine stimulant Cylert (pemoline). The nine children displayed the following "psychotic symptoms":

1. Bizarre behavior
2. Paranoia
3. Visual hallucinations
4. Auditory hallucinations; aggressive, agitated behavior
5. Unrealistic fear of being harmed by other children
6. Bizarre behavior, giddiness
7. Depression, hallucinations, suicidal behavior
8. Euphoria, flight of ideas, decreased sleep, increased energy
9. Concrete thought [a sign of psychosis or brain disfunction], severe depression

Not all of these descriptions necessarily fit the category of psychosis; the severity apparently led to their inclusion in the chart. Note the wide range of these reactions, including paranoia and aggression, depression and suicidality, and manic-like euphoria. This broad spectrum is consistent with the literature on stimulants and my own clinical experience.

These severe reactions developed in children across an age range from four to seventeen. They occurred as early in the treatment as the first or second dose (three cases) or as long after the start of treatment as seven years (one case). Two of the nine cases (numbers 1 and 6 above) occurred after only one 5-mg dose of Ritalin. Many physicians have no idea that psychiatric drugs often cause severe abnormal mental reactions after the first dose or two.

Most—but not all—of the symptoms cleared up when the stimulant medication was stopped. Of course, ADHD-like behaviors are not usually associated with psychosis. The few children who failed to recover were probably driven into chronic psychosis by the medications.

Causing Zombie-Like and Robotic Behavior

Robotic and depressed behaviors in children are very similar and overlapping. A child who is depressed will also lack self-motivation and self-worth and feel unable to make choices. This can create a robot-like docility that's likely to be punctuated by outbursts of resistance.

Some experts in the field, for example, Peter Jensen, have publicly dismissed the idea that children can be made zombie-like by prescribed stimulants. Yet in the less public forum of a chapter in a widely read psychiatric textbook, Jensen himself and his coauthor describe the zombie effect and mention it by name.

Jensen and his coauthor make a remarkable admission in their chapter in the textbook. Talking about children treated with stimulants, they describe "the amphetamine look, a pinched, somber expression."[11] They go on to say that it is "harmless in itself but worrisome to parents, who can be reassured." But what kind of doctor would so cavalierly dismiss a "pinched, somber expression" in a child? Jensen and his coauthor then discuss "the behavioral equivalent" of this amphetamine look. They call it "the 'zombie' constriction of affect [feeling] and spontaneity." This zombie effect is related to the overall tendency of stimulants to cause depression. The authors themselves observe that stimulants can cause "depression, rarely with suicidal ideation."

The zombie effect in children occurs along a continuum. In relatively mild expressions, their eyes lose their sparkle and their personalities lose their edge. Their spirit seems dampened; their responses are less spontaneous. But only someone who knows and loves them, someone who is "in touch" with them, might notice. "My child just didn't seem like himself anymore. I hardly knew him," parents have often told me. Often they will add, "Sure, he was easier to be around, but it made me sad, because I'd lost him in the process."

Causing Obsessive-Compulsive Behavior

Most children taking stimulants will become abnormally obsessive and compulsive in their behavior. A study conducted at NIMH[12] found that more than half of the children treated with stimulants develop signs of drug-induced obsessive-compulsive disorder. In some cases, it can be very severe, such as in the case of a child who raked leaves for seven straight hours and then waited for individual leaves to fall off the trees. More often, the children persisted at games or other activities in a compulsive, unending fashion. They would bear down too hard on their pencils, repetitively erase, or spend too much time worrying over details. Even a single dose can make children overfocus on tasks of little intrinsic merit or interest, even to the point that it will be difficult to stop them.[13]

Why don't most doctors and researchers recognize such frequent harmful stimulant effects? First, they don't want to see them and don't look for them. Second, when they notice them, they tend to consider them improvements. The children seem to be more obedient and to be working harder. Third, when the obsessive or compulsive symptoms become very severe, they blame them on the child's "emerging obsessive-compulsive disorder" rather than on the drug.

Reconfirming How Stimulants Really Work

Primarily through discussion of animal studies, Chapter 3 showed that stimulants suppress all spontaneous behavior and enforce submissive and obsessive-compulsive behavior. We have now confirmed the same effects in children. These suppressive effects are the primary or so-called therapeutic effect of the drugs. That is, the drugs work precisely by suppressing the mental life and behavior of the children, making them more docile and easier to manage and making them more willing to focus on boring or resented tasks.

Table 3.1 (in Chapter 3), entitled "Harmful Stimulant Drug Reactions Commonly Misidentified as 'Therapeutic' or 'Beneficial,'" is drawn from a review of twenty controlled clinical trials involving children treated for ADHD with Ritalin or Dexedrine (amphetamine). We can expect very similar if not identical effects from any of the commonly used stimulants. This table demonstrates the wide range of suppressive effects commonly reported in clinical studies. Once again, these are not really side effects, they are primary effects; they make the drugs work.

Lessons from Overdose

It is worth reemphasizing the point made in Table 4.1: A great deal can be revealed about a drug's effects from examining the known results of overdosing. Effects that might go unnoticed at lower doses become amplified during overdose, providing insight into what might be happening in more sensitive people during routine dosing.

The example of the mild stimulant caffeine can be helpful in this regard. Some people become anxious, agitated, and irritable after a single cup of coffee. I have seen patients react to the amount of caffeine that remains in some decaffeinated coffees. On the other hand, some people can drink several mugs of coffee without becoming anxious, agitated, or irritable. Overall, however, the tendency of caffeine to produce these harmful stimulating effects will become more apparent with increasing dose and ultimately with overdose in people who drink much too much coffee.

The label for Adderall XR admits the very point that I am making. Under "Overdosage," it states the following: *"Individual patient response to amphetamines varies widely. Toxic symptoms may occur idiosyncratically at low doses."*

I have written the above quote in italics for emphasis. Parents, patients, and prescribing physicians should emblazon that warning on their minds.

What are the "toxic symptoms" that may occur "at low doses"? The following description is provided in the Adderall XR label:

> Manifestations of acute overdosage with amphetamines include restlessness, tremor, hyperreflexia, rapid respiration, confusion, assaultiveness, hallucinations, panic state, hyperpyrexia [very high fever] and rhabdomyolysis [severe destruction of muscle]. Fatigue and depression usually follow the central nervous system stimulation. Cardiovascular effects include arrhythmias, hypertension or hypotension and circulatory collapse. Gastrointestinal symptoms include nausea, vomiting, diarrhea, and abdominal cramps. Fatal poisoning is usually preceded by convulsions and coma.

The warning that individual responses vary widely and that "toxic symptoms" can occur at "low doses" directly precedes this list of symptoms of overdose. As this book confirms, these symptoms of overdose can and do occur at the lower doses routinely used to treat children and adults.

Stimulants are dangerous drugs. Giving them to children is a kind of Russian roulette with pills. The existence of such high rates of serious psychiatric adverse reactions indicates that stimulant drugs cause underlying brain malfunctions. Chapter 5 will address these stimulant-induced malfunctions.

How Stimulants Harm
the Child's Brain

Earlier chapters documented the wide range of abnormal mental or psychiatric reactions caused by the stimulants. Many of them occur along the stimulant continuum that begins with milder insomnia, tension, or irritability and can progress to mania and psychosis with aggression. They can cause gross impairments of brain function, including delirium, confusion, and convulsions. The stimulants can also paradoxically cause depression and lethargy. Tables 3.1 and 4.1–4.3 summarize these adverse psychiatric and neurological effects from various perspectives, including their high rates of occurrence.

Why would drugs like Ritalin, Focalin, Concerta, Dexedrine, and Adderall produce so many harmful effects on the mind? The answer is: because they harm the brain.

Research continues to confirm that all of the stimulants have similar effects on the brain, including Ritalin, Focalin, Concerta, Adderall, Dexedrine, and Desoxyn, as well as cocaine. Recent findings from state-of-the-art brain imaging techniques led to a recent headline in the *Journal of the American Medical Association*:[1] "Pay attention: Ritalin acts much like cocaine."

TABLE 5.1   Stimulant-Induced Brain Damage and Dysfunction Demonstrated in Human and Animal Research

Reduced blood flow
Reduced oxygen supply
Reduced energy utilization
Persistent biochemical imbalances
Persistent loss of receptors for neurotransmitters
Persistent sensitization (increased reactivity to stimulants)
Permanent distortion of brain cell structure and function
Brain cell death and tissue shrinkage

This chapter will review the harmful effects on the brain produced by stimulant drugs. As in most scientific literature, there are conflicting reports. However, all of the effects listed in Table 5.1 have been demonstrated in well-conducted animal and human research, often in relatively short-term studies using drug doses that equal or do not far exceed those routinely used in the treatment of children. Shrinkage of areas of the brain, for example, has been shown in children exposed to routine treatment with stimulant drugs including amphetamines (Adderall, Dexedrine) and methylphenidate (Ritalin).

Gross Malfunctions with the First Dose

From the first dose, stimulants cause gross malfunctions in the brain. That's how and why they work so quickly. Researchers at the Brookhaven National Laboratory gave routine doses of Ritalin to normal volunteers. Much like cocaine, Ritalin reduced the blood flow 23–30 percent in all areas of the brain, including the frontal lobes, where the highest human functions are generated. The changes were so gross that they were apparent on brain-scan photographs printed in a scientific journal.[2]

When blood flow is reduced to any portion of the body, including the brain, it causes the organ to receive less oxygen and less nutrition, resulting in an overall loss of function. Researchers at NIMH's Laboratory of Cerebral Metabolism found that Ritalin reduced the gross metabolic rate "throughout many portions of the brain" in animals.[3] In other words, many parts of the brain stopped functioning at their normal level of activity. As the researchers pointed out, these pharmacological changes would occur in any animal or person, whether or not the individual had ADHD-like behaviors.

What happens when the blood flow, oxygen, and nutrition are reduced to any organ of the body? It causes the organ to malfunction. For example, when blood flow is reduced to your heart, it eventually causes heart failure.

When your child seems to become quieter and even "more content" after the first dose of any stimulant drug, your child is in effect suffering from a discernible degree of "brain failure." With less brain function, your child is less spontaneous and demanding.

Can these gross changes lead to permanent damage? The brain, especially the brain of a child, is a vulnerable organ. At the least, we must be concerned that gross suppression of blood flow, oxygenation, and nutrition would lead to damage.

Unfortunately, there have been few systematic attempts to investigate irreversible brain damage caused by these medications. The drug companies sponsor most research in the field and often control what gets published.[4] Nonetheless, there are plenty of indications that these drugs can cause permanent harm.

The Vulnerability of the Brain to Damage

There are more than 100 billion neurons (brain cells) in the brain. These are supported and controlled by untold billions of other cells that create the matrix of the brain. Each of the billions of neurons has as many as 10,000 or more connections to other cells. The result is a complex organ with trillions of interconnections.

Every individual human brain is more complex than the entire physical universe. Astrophysics is kid stuff compared to the study of one person's brain function. Life, in essence, is enormously more complicated than the material universe.

Considering the complexity and vulnerability of the brain with its infinitely fine-tuned operations, it is obviously risky to introduce essentially toxic foreign substances into it. Meanwhile, there's pitifully little research concerning the potential harm done to the brain by stimulant drugs. However, what we know is sufficient to warn us against bathing the growing brains of children in these substances.

Disrupting the Brain's Normal Biochemical Balances

Stimulant drugs "rev up," or overactivate, at least three neurotransmitters or chemical messengers—dopamine, norepinephrine, and serotonin. These neurotransmitter networks reach into every nook and cranny of the brain, affecting most of its functions. Disrupting any of these large, complex pathways would be sufficient to endanger the proper function, growth, and development of a child's brain; disrupting all three at once is a prescription for disaster. I have described these harmful effects in detail in *Talking Back to Ritalin* (rev. ed., 2001a) and in my scientific publications in professional journals.[5] What follows is an abbreviated summary.

When stimulants cause neurotransmitter systems to become overactive, the systems try to compensate by shutting down. The brain tries to reduce the impact of the overactivity in its neurotransmitter systems. When the drugs are removed, these compensatory mechanisms cause rebound and withdrawal problems, and can lead to abuse and addiction.

The brain is injured directly by the toxic effects of the drugs and indirectly by the brain's own attempts to compensate for the toxicity. Animal experiments indicate that both the direct and indirect effects can become persistent and even permanent.

Some of the most commonly used stimulants, including Dexedrine and Adderall, are pure amphetamine. Amphetamines have been shown to cause permanent structural abnormalities in .the brains of animals at clinical doses administered for only five days a week for a five-week period. In one study, cells in the frontal lobes became irreversibly deformed.[6] The frontal lobes are the center of all higher human functions, including impulsive control, thinking, judgment, and abstract reasoning.

Another study used brain-scan methods to study the effect of two relatively small doses of amphetamine on the brains of monkeys. It found changes in brain-chemistry function lasting several months or more.[7] In a similar study using larger doses over a period of ten days, the investigators found that amphetamine produced signs of "neurotoxicity" lasting two years, until the termination of the project.[8]

Methamphetamine under the trade name Desoxyn is prescribed for children diagnosed with ADHD. This is, of course, the same psychoactive substance that is notorious for abuse as a street drug. Animal research has documented severe brain damage from methamphetamine, including the massive death of brain cells.[9] It is astonishing that the FDA allows this drug to be prescribed for children. Unfortunately, Ritalin is so closely related to methamphetamine, as well as to amphetamine, that it becomes extremely likely that Ritalin is also producing irreversible damage and cell death, even if to a somewhat lesser degree.

There are fewer studies on the impact of methylphenidate (Ritalin) on the brain. Thus far, the harmful effects measured on a neuronal and biochemical level seem to be more short-lived; that is, the brain may recuperate from the most obvious damage over a period of weeks or months. Some biochemical changes seem to be more persistent, including heightened sensitivity to later doses of the drug. However, there is little comfort in the failure of the more sparse Ritalin studies to show the same extensive damage as found with amphetamine (Adderall, Dexedrine) and methamphetamine. Studies showing atrophy to various parts of the brains of children treated with Ritalin confirm that Ritalin also causes permanent damage to the brain (see below).

In fact, as our methods of studying brain function become more refined, I am confident they will reconfirm that stimulants produce irreversible harm to the brain. There are two relatively recent examples of this.

In December 1999, researchers at Harvard Medical School found an increase in the number (density) of a chemical transporter in the brains of children diagnosed with ADHD.[10] The transporter removes one of the neurotransmitters—dopamine—from the active space between neurons (the synapses). *The researchers specifically required that the participating children be taken off stimulant drugs for thirty days prior to the study.* This confirms that at least some of the children (and perhaps most or all) had prior exposure to stimulants.

What is the likely cause of this increased density of the system that removes dopamine from the synapses? It is almost certainly a compensatory mechanism that the brain uses to overcome increased drug-induced hyperactivity of dopamine. Stimulants not only increase the output of dopamine into the synapse, they block the removal by the transporter system. By increasing the "muscle" of the transporter, the brain tries to overcome the stimulant effects.

In a sad commentary on the bias of drug advocates, these researchers completely fail to note that the abnormality was almost certainly due to stimulants. Instead, they attribute it to ADHD. Since the children had been taken off the drugs one month earlier, it indicates a chronic drug-induced abnormality.

Confirming my interpretation of the study, recent brain-scan studies have shown that Ritalin is a more potent blocker of the transporter system than cocaine.[11] This means that Ritalin will force the transporter system into an unusually vigorous effort to compensate for the blocking.

Even more recently, an as yet unpublished paper by scientists at the University of Buffalo was presented at the annual meeting of the Society for Neuroscientists.[12] Joan Baizer, Ph.D., senior author of the study and professor of physiology and biophysics, made the following observations:

Clinicians consider Ritalin to be short-acting. When the active dose has worked its way through the system, they consider it "all gone." Our research with gene expression in an animal model suggests it has the potential for causing long-lasting changes in brain cell structure and function.

Baizer compared these findings on Ritalin to research already carried out in regard to amphetamine and cocaine.

Everett Ellinwood, M.D., is professor of psychiatry and pharmacology at the Duke University Medical Center and one of the most experienced researchers in the field. Based on the existing scientific literature, he concluded that the doses of stimulants used to treat children have been proven to cause persistent damage in animals: "Drug levels in children on a mg/kg basis are sometimes as high as those reported to produce chronic CNS [central nervous system] changes in animal studies."[13] Another experienced researcher described these changes as "damage to cerebral blood vessels, neuronal loss and microhemorrhages."[14]

Causing Future Supersensitivity to Stimulants

Many carefully conducted animal experiments have indicated yet another kind of long-term harm done to the brain by stimulants. Relatively low-dose short-term exposure to stimulants in monkeys causes a persistent sensitization to the drug. Low doses administered at a later date will produce an unusually strong behavioral and biochemical reaction. That is, the drugs create a biochemical dysfunction characterized by a supersensitivity to further doses of the stimulant. The stimulant doses used in the monkey experiments have been relatively small and brief, but the sensitization changes were long-lasting and probably permanent.[15] Following only twelve weeks of low-dose exposure to amphetamine, *the sensitization effects lasted for more than three and one-half years.*[16]

These long-lasting and probably permanent effects were measured in two ways: first, by evaluating the animal's behavioral response at a later time to a single new dose of amphetamine and, second, by using advanced brain imaging techniques to measure persistent biochemical changes in the brain.

The behavioral changes involved the same kind of stimulant-induced responses described in the animal experiments in Chapter 3, such as drug-induced compulsive or stereotypical behaviors. The biochemical changes involved an increased tendency for the stimulant to cause the release of the neurotransmitter dopamine.

These studies should be viewed as containing an extremely important warning: Even relatively short-term exposure to stimulants can cause long-term and probably irreversible changes in the brain. Is this change good for the brain? Not likely. It is an impairment, however subtle, that will likely remain with the child for life.

We don't know the overall impact of stimulant drugs on the growth and development of the child, or on the child's future capacities, and it will be difficult to measure these negative consequences. However, we do know that this sensitization is likely to produce an increased responsiveness to all kinds of stimulants later in life, including Ritalin, amphetamine, methamphetamine, and cocaine. This is probably one of the mechanisms by which treatment with stimulants for ADHD increases cocaine abuse in young adulthood (Chapter 7).

Research on Humans Confirms
Brain Damage from Ritalin

It's known that stimulant addicts can develop permanent brain damage. In regard to stimulants prescribed to children by doctors, one study has demonstrated shrinkage in the brains of adults who were exposed during childhood to stimulants such as Ritalin.[17] It is, of course, far more likely that the damage was done by the drugs rather than by "ADHD."

Similarly, multiple studies have demonstrated a variety of brain abnormalities in children diagnosed with ADHD; but it turns out that these studies have involved children exposed to stimulants and often to multiple psychiatric drugs. The great number of studies indicating "differences" in the brains of children diagnosed with ADHD in fact confirms the damaging effects of stimulant medications on the growing child's brain.[18]

At the November 1998 Consensus Development Conference on the Diagnosis and Treatment of Attention Deficit Hyperactivity Disorder, James Swanson presented data supposedly confirming the biological basis of ADHD. He showed brain scans displaying a variety of inconsistent changes in the brains of children diagnosed with ADHD, including shrinkage of various areas of the brain. Only when challenged did he belatedly admit that *all* of the studies involved children who had been treated with stimulants and often with many other psychiatric drugs. This included highly touted studies conducted at the NIMH.[19]

There was, of course, no scientific justification for Swanson or any other doctor claiming that the damage in the children's brains was due to "ADHD" rather than the drugs. However, there *is* a scientific basis for attributing the damage to the drugs, since we know that stimulants grossly impair brain function and can cause permanent microscopic and biochemical damage. Brain-scan studies showing abnormalities in the brains of children diagnosed with ADHD and treated with stimulants should be taken as further confirmation that stimulant drugs can produce gross brain damage. Tragically, they are used instead to promote the drugging of children.

It seems inevitable that exposing a child's brain to stimulants for months at a time will result in permanent malfunctions of the child's brain. Since the mental and behavioral manifestations will be largely indistinguishable from possible developmental and psychological problems, it will be difficult to pin them down with any certainty. Unfortunately, this has given free rein to those doctors who prefer to make false claims that the drugs are harmless to the brain and mind.

Increased Risk to the Brain from Sustained-Release Stimulants

There is an especially ominous aspect to the increasing use of long-acting preparations such as Concerta and Adderall XR. Studies of brain damage from amphetamine exposure have found that "prolonged plasma levels are more crucial in producing neurotoxicity than higher but more transient plasma levels." The researchers opine, "Apparently neuronal systems have developed more effective ways to cope with sudden and brief insults than with progressive, more prolonged ones."[20]

Although not noted by the researchers, nor published by anyone else until now, their observations should raise very serious concerns about the relatively greater neurotoxicity of the newer sustained-release stimulant preparations.[21] All of them aim at providing a more constant serum level of the stimulant drug. Because they impose a steady level of drug on the brain, the brain has less opportunity to bounce back or recover. *As a result, Concerta, Metadate ER, Ritalin SR, Methylin SR, and Adderall XR are likely to produce more harm to the brain than their shorter-acting versions.*

Stimulants pose additional risks to the brain in the form of internal bleeding, inflammation of the blood vessels, and stroke. These will be dealt with in Chapter 6.

In summary, stimulants cause gross malfunctions in the brain with the very first dose, accounting for their immediate subduing effect on the behavior of children. Exposure to repeated doses of stimulants in animals over a period of days or a few weeks can cause persistent or permanent damage to their brains. Most disturbing, multiple brain-scan studies of children diagnosed with ADHD and treated with stimulants, including Ritalin, have shown shrinkage in a variety of areas of the brain. This damage is most logically attributed to the stimulant drugs. It is caused by their well-documented adverse effects on the brain.

How Stimulants
Harm the Child's Body

Chapters 3–5 described harmful stimulant effects on mental life, behavior, and the brain. From the heart to the skin, stimulants can also harm a variety of other organs of the body. By interfering with normal growth-hormone production, stimulants impair and even stunt the growth of the entire body.

Some harmful effects on the body result indirectly from the disruption of brain function, some result more directly from toxic effects on the organs themselves, and some result from both.

Stimulants, for example, can overtax the heart by causing an elevated heart rate and hypertension. The changes occur from overstimulating the sympathetic portion of the autonomic nervous system. At the same time, stimulants can weaken the heart through a direct toxic effect on cardiac muscle. The combination can be deadly.

Overall, the stimulants have many serious adverse physical effects. Table 4.1 in Chapter 4 lists toxic reactions to the drug as disclosed in the FDA-approved labels. Table 4.2 in Chapter 4 provides a summary overview of adverse effects caused by the stimulants, including ones that are primarily manifested physically.

Remember, an adverse effect produced by one kind of stimulant such as Ritalin, Concerta, or Metadate SR can usually be produced by the other stimulants as well, including Dexedrine and Adderall.

Stunting Growth

In many cases, the growth of children is obviously suppressed or even stunted by stimulants. Some of the children look skinny and unhealthy as if starving, while others seem normal. Most will rebound with an unbelievably rapid growth in height and weight—if the drugs are stopped while the child is still growing. In one study, Ritalin reduced the expected monthly weight gain by 25 percent.[1] When the drug was stopped, weight gain accelerated far above the normally expected rate.

When children seem to be growing well while taking stimulants, some doctors or parents will observe, "John's very big; the stimulants haven't hurt him." Unfortunately, we don't know how tall or large Johnny might have become without the drug, and the fact that he's achieved an even above-average size says little about the drug's actual effect on his unique genetic endowment for growth.

Too many doctors are misled into believing that growth suppression is a relatively harmless problem that results from a child losing his or her appetite. However, there's more to it than the mere loss of appetite. The stimulants cause marked dysfunction in the production of growth hormone. Specifically, they cause an abnormal increase in growth hormone during the day and then an abnormal compensatory suppression of the hormone at night, when it most significantly affects growth.

The impact on growth hormone is so dramatic that researchers have observed that growth-hormone levels can be used as a marker for whether or not children are taking their medication. If the growth-hormone cycle isn't disrupted, then the children are not taking the medication. Because stimulants always impair growth-hormone production, we should assume that there is always some impairment of growth, even if it remains grossly undetectable.[2]

Some doctors used to tell parents not to worry about growth suppression because there is a compensatory growth spurt when the drugs are stopped. While the body does try to catch up when the stimulant is stopped, the phase of accelerated growth is abnormally rapid and not necessarily altogether healthy. In addition, there's no guarantee that irreversible harm hasn't been done along the way during weeks or months of stimulant treatment. Furthermore, nowadays children are kept on stimulants for months or years at a time, so the body is given no opportunity to go through a growth spurt.

The disruption of growth hormone should be viewed as an ominous finding. It means that all growth processes are being impaired, including the growth of the brain, heart, and lungs. The entire body relies on growth hormone to regulate its developmental processes. Citing many research reports, a respected research team wrote:

> Research reveals that methylphenidate stimulates daytime release of growth hormone, disrupting the usual nocturnal release. This is troublesome since disturbances in the normal release of growth hormone may not only influence height velocity but may also impair other critical aspects of physical development such as sexual maturation.[3]

The researchers should also have emphasized the threat to the growth of the brain and hence the mind.

The authors of a medical textbook suggest that the growth lag caused by stimulants is temporary "in most cases."[4] This assumes that the children are given regular drug vacations in order to catch up. Although these authors are staunch advocates of stimulants for children, they go on to recognize that "the effects on growth that the long-term use of stimulants has on children leads some physicians to believe that this drug should never be prescribed for children." This observation—like many others in this book—should give strength to parents who believe, as I do, that children should never be given these drugs for "ADHD" or the control of behavior.

Despite decades of sophisticated research demonstrating that stimulants disrupt growth hormone, cause growth suppression, and lead to accelerated growth spurts when stopped, some drug advocates have tried to demonstrate that there are no significant effects on growth. In my experience, the doctors who make these claims typically go to extremes in order to convince professionals and parents that it's safe to use these drugs. One such study was published in 1996 in an attempt to undermine a large, consistent body of research demonstrating growth suppression.[5] However, the new study used only one measurement of height and weight for each child and attempted to draw conclusions from it. The researchers did not use consecutive measures on the same child to show the effect of the drug; they took one measure on every child and attempted to compare that one measurement to a similar measure in a control group of children who were not drug treated. Using these dubious methods as well as a badly flawed control group and questionable statistics, the authors leaped from one single measurement to a conclusion about the long-term effect of stimulants on growth. By contrast, many other studies have used multiple measurements to show a definite inhibition of growth.

As a result of disrupting pituitary function, stimulants also interfere with the normal cycles of prolactin production. Prolactin can be found throughout the body, but its functions are poorly understood. It does, however, participate in the regulation of sexual development, yet another fact that should raise caution in regard to giving stimulants to children and adolescents.

Causing Heart Problems

As already noted, stimulants produce a combined assault on the heart, first by overstimulating heart rate and blood pressure, and then by weakening the muscles of the overstressed organ. Palpitations are one signal that the heart is beating irregularly.

What's the result?

My review of spontaneous reports of adverse Ritalin effects made to the FDA disclosed a very large number of Ritalin-induced cases of cardiovascular disease.[6] Many concerned the well-known problem of stimulant-caused hypertension. Most of them involved arrhythmias and conduction problems that sometimes cause sudden cardiac arrest. There were more than a dozen reports of cardiac arrest or heart failure. This was a relatively small portion of the 2,821 reports made during the period of time (1985 through early 1997) but presents an important signal of danger.

I have been consulted in several cases in which stimulant drugs have caused fatal cardiac arrhythmias in children. In one case, the child's heart on autopsy showed a pattern of deterioration that the coroner compared to changes he had observed in chronic cocaine addicts.

A number of animal studies confirm that stimulants such as Ritalin weaken heart muscle and reduce its function.[7] Stimulants also cause high blood pressure, a special concern among African-American boys, who are especially prone to develop severe hypertension as relatively young adults.[8] Weakened heart muscle combined with hypertension is, of course, a hazard for any human being.

Causing Strokes

Ritalin, Adderall, and all stimulants can cause strokes (cerebral vascular accidents). These potentially catastrophic events can result from bleeding or inflammation of the blood vessels in the brain. Hypertension probably plays a key role in many of these disasters. Physicians sometimes seem particularly unaware of stimulant-induced strokes, probably leading to underreporting of the problem.

Bleeding in the brain in association with oral amphetamine use has been reported in the literature since 1970. There are reports of strokes after a "single low dose exposure," but most reports have been made in association with stimulant abuse.[9]

A report in *Lancet* in 1988 described the first published case of stroke involving Ritalin in a boy receiving the drug for hyperactivity.[10] The author observed, "Physicians who prescribe methylphenidate [Ritalin] for long-term use should be aware of this potential complication and specifically question patients regarding symptoms of cerebral ischaemia [reduced blood flow], including headache." Remember that Ritalin and amphetamine both produce gross reductions in blood flow to the brain, thereby creating the conditions for stroke.

A report in 2000 in the *Journal of Child Neurology* describes the case of an eight-year-old boy who developed vasculitis and stroke after taking Ritalin for one and one-half years for hyperactivity.[11] These authors also issue a warning: "We draw your attention to the risk of using methylphenidate [Ritalin] for a long period of time."

Overall, stimulants pose serious cardiovascular hazards. Individuals suffering from or at risk of experiencing hypertension, heart disease, or strokes should especially avoid stimulants.

Beware Ephedra

The stimulants are causing far more heart problems than are currently recognized. The medical profession and the FDA are far more eager to focus on the adverse effects of "alternative" treatments. In recent years, a great deal of attention has been given to the hazards of ephedra, a 5,000-year-old Chinese herbal remedy that has stimulant properties. Ephedra is by no means as powerful as Ritalin or amphetamine, but its widespread use as an alternative to these drugs has drawn fire from the medical establishment. The *Washington Post* summarized the dangers associated with ephedra:[12]

Increased blood pressure and heart rate, insomnia, heart attack and stroke. Instances of mania, psychosis and seizures have also been reported. Between 1993 and 1996, the FDA collected nearly 700 reports of adverse reactions and thirty-nine deaths.

The above summary should look familiar to anyone who has gotten this far in this book. Every one of the listed adverse effects can occur with Ritalin, Adderall, or any other stimulant. If we gave as much attention to the hazards of prescribed stimulants, we would find their adverse effects to be far more frequent and dangerous than those associated with ephedra. It is hypocritical for experts and the FDA to focus so much attention on ephedra while ignoring the even more dangerous prescription stimulants.

Causing Tics

Stimulant drugs commonly produce tics (involuntary twitching).[13] Many cases have been reported to the FDA, I have evaluated numerous cases, and there are many studies of the problem in the literature. Several controlled clinical trials have demonstrated a high rate of stimulant-induced tics and nervous movements in children. One trial found a fourfold increase in tics in children treated with Ritalin. Altogether 12.5 percent developed tics and about one-fourth of these were serious.[14] Another clinical trial found that 58 percent of their children developed tics on Ritalin and Dexedrine, with one that was apparently irreversible.[15] While the figures vary enormously, all clinical trials that look for tics find that a large percentage of children developed them during stimulant treatment.

There have also been a number of retrospective chart reviews aimed at determining the rate of stimulant-induced tics. These reviews rely on clinical observations by treating physicians rather than on data generated in more closely watched clinical trials. Therefore, they are much less likely to observe and/or to record the tics. Nonetheless, they also confirm that stimulants cause tics.

One retrospective study of 122 children found that 9 percent developed tics, including one severe irreversible case with "facial twitching, head turning, lip smacking, forehead wiping, and vocalizations."[16] Another retrospective study of 555 subjects in three different clinics found a rate of approximately 8 percent for the development of tics.[17] In keeping with good standards of practice, the clinics excluded from stimulant treatment any children with a prior history of tics and stopped the medication immediately upon discovering the emergence of tics. Therefore, the rates were lower than would be anticipated in less-disciplined clinical situations. The rate of 8 percent was roughly the same for Ritalin, amphetamine, and Cylert (pemoline). Younger children were more susceptible to developing drug-induced tics.

The Ritalin label warns doctors not to prescribe Ritalin to children who have tics or have a family history of tics. The Adderall XR label has a similar but weaker precaution.

Too many physicians ignore these warning with disastrous, tragic results. I have consulted in several cases in which doctors ignored the warning signs and the youngster developed permanent disfiguring tics of the face or neck.

I have also seen cases in which physicians have used antipsychotic medications such as Mellaril, Haldol, or Risperdal to suppress children's tics that were originally caused by stimulant drug treatment. They have done this without fully apprising the parents of the extreme danger that the antipsychotic drugs would permanently worsen the tics while temporarily suppressing them (discussed in Chapter 2). Probably because the children were already suffering from stimulant damage to the region of the brain that controls movement, these children rapidly developed severe, permanent tics while on the antipsychotics.

Causing Convulsions

Seizures come in many forms. At one extreme, grand mal convulsions cause people to fall into unconsciousness while their limbs go into spasms. But there are more subtle kinds of seizures that can result in little more than a brief lapse of attention or a staring into space from which the individual quickly recovers with little or no recognition of what has happened.

Seizures result from overactivity of one or more areas of the brain, causing a disorganized firing of neurons. Sedatives tend to reduce or control seizures by slowing down or quieting the brain. By the opposite process, stimulants can cause seizures. They can also increase the risk of further seizures in individuals who are already prone to them. The drug label for Ritalin warns about the possible production of seizures, and numerous reports of seizures in association with stimulants have been made to the FDA.[18]

Causing Gastrointestinal Problems

Stimulants commonly cause gastrointestinal problems. While this is well known to doctors, the range of these problems is greater than usually thought, including stomachaches, cramps, nausea, constipation, diarrhea, dryness and a bad taste in the mouth, and abnormal liver functions.

My review of FDA reports concerning Ritalin disclosed a surprising number pertaining to liver malfunction. The 2001 Ritalin label mentions isolated cases of coma due to hepatic malfunction in association with Ritalin.

Causing Headaches and Blurred Vision

Headaches are another well-known adverse effect of stimulants. Blurred vision is another drug-induced problem that can be mistaken for poor concentration or other ADHD-like symptoms.

Causing Hair Loss and Hair Pulling

Doctors are less likely to recognize that stimulants can cause hair loss. Hair loss, of course, can be especially humiliating and disfiguring for children. In addition, some children taking stimulants will obsessively pull out their hair, even denuding their eyebrows or scalps.

Causing Skin and Joint Disorders

Skin rashes can also occur. On rare occasions they can become severe and life threatening, sometimes as a part of dangerous hypersensitivity reactions that involve other organs of the body.[19] These reactions may include one or more of the following: hives, peeling skin, large irregular blotches, bleeding into the skin, joint pain, and fever.

Causing Blood Disorders

My review of reports to the FDA disclosed a surprisingly large number concerning suppression of the white blood-cell count (leukopenia). The Ritalin label mentions leukopenia, thrombocytopenia, and anemia. Leukopenia can cause weakened resistance to infection. Thrombocytopenia is the loss of blood platelets necessary for clotting and leads to bleeding into the skin and other organs of the body. Anemia, of course, can cause weakness, fatigue, and other difficulties.

Children taking stimulants should regularly have their blood tested, including liver function tests, platelet counts, and complete blood counts.

Causing Sexual Dysfunction

Stimulants can cause impotence and other abnormalities in sexual behavior as a direct drug effect and as a result of interfering with the quality of emotional relationships.

Risks During Pregnancy and Nursing

Stimulants should not be used during pregnancy or nursing. They cross the placenta and impair the fetus. They also enter mother's milk and harm the newborn. In addition, stimulant-induced disruption of prolactin production in the mother may interfere with the mother's physical capacity to nurse.

The Adderall label correctly warns: "Infants born to mothers dependent on amphetamine have an increased risk of premature delivery and low birth weight. Also, these infants may experience symptoms of withdrawal as demonstrated by dysphoria, including agitation, and significant lassitude." There is also a potential risk of malformations in the newborn.

The official label for the new long-acting amphetamine Adderall XR contains a particularly detailed warning about using stimulants during pregnancy. It states that rodents exposed to clinical doses of amphetamine during the prenatal and early postnatal period have developed "long-term neurochemical and behavior alterations." These included "learning and memory deficits," altered activity levels, and changes in sexual functions.[20]

Liver Tumors

Ritalin has been found to produce a rare liver tumor in mice, causing the FDA to require a precautions statement in the label. The actual research was surrounded with controversy. The FDA itself labeled the finding a "weak signal." The researchers themselves were split on this issue. One of the three researchers proposed to the FDA panel that the cancer findings be declared a "clear signal." It was defeated by a 4–3 vote with two abstentions. As in most places in psychiatric drug research, politics seemed to be at work.[21]

Neuroleptic Malignant Syndrome

The 2001 Ritalin label mentions "very rare reports of neuroleptic malignant syndrome (NMS)." NMS is an extraordinarily devastating, potentially fatal disorder. It has been of special interest to me because it is a well-established but commonly overlooked adverse reaction to neuroleptic drugs such as Mellaril, Prolixin, Haldol, Risperdal, and Zyprexa.[22] NMS is easily confused with viral encephalitis of the brain. It causes severe mental changes and possibly coma, severe abnormal movements, fever, blood pressure and cardiac dysfunction, and other symptoms. The potential for Ritalin and other stimulants to cause NMS remains controversial.

Dangerous Interactions with Other Drugs

Stimulants interact dangerously with a number of medications. In combination with monoamine oxidase inhibitors (MAOI) antidepressants such as Nardil and Parnate, they can cause severe hypertension and/or fever and death. In fact, any antidepressant becomes more dangerous in combination with stimulants, potentially increasing the risk of many adverse reactions including mania, psychosis, seizures, and cardiovascular problems. Problems can also occur in combination with some cold and allergy medications that contain mild stimulants (sympathomimetic amines).

When the stomach is alkaline rather than acidic, there is *increased absorption* of stimulants. This can dangerously elevate the stimulant blood level. Therefore, anyone taking stimulants should avoid taking stomach and digestive aids that counteract the acidity of the stomach, including antacids like Tums or Rolaids.

A variety of drugs will either increase or decrease the effects of stimulants. Anyone anticipating using these drugs should review the drug interactions section of the label in the *Physicians' Desk Reference* or another detailed source.

Worsening Preexisting Conditions

Avoid using stimulants if you have glaucoma, any kind of cardiovascular disorder, arteriosclerosis (including "hardening of the arteries"), even borderline hypertension, prostatic hypertrophy, or hyperthyroidism. Stimulants can interfere with drugs used to treat these disorders and worsen the disorders themselves.

As the labels for stimulants confirm, individuals who have severe emotional disturbances, including depression and psychosis, should especially avoid these drugs. Stimulants such as Adderall and Ritalin can worsen these psychiatric problems.

Use in Very Young Children

Stimulants for ADHD are not FDA-approved for children under age six. While these drugs are dangerous to children of any age, they are especially hazardous for the very young. First, there are the dangers of disrupting the normal growth and development of the brain. Second, there is the more subtle risk of suppressing overall spontaneity during periods of personal and educational growth. Then there is the known increase in the rate and severity of adverse emotional reactions in younger children treated with stimulants.

A controlled clinical trial of Ritalin given to children age four to six disclosed enormous rates of serious adverse effects.[23] For example, 69 percent of the children were markedly deteriorated in regard to becoming more unhappy and sad, and 62 percent were similarly deteriorated in regard to becoming less interested in others. Severe symptoms increased 12 percent for "Uninterested in others" and 28 percent for "Talks less with others." Nightmares increased 35 percent, and tics or nervous movements increased 9 percent.

It is shameful that the National Institute of Mental Health (NIMH), in effect acting as an arm of the pharmaceutical industry, is currently conducting further clinical trials on children age two to six. The trials should be stopped.

The Extra Hazard of Long-Acting (Sustained-Release) Preparations

Stimulant preparations vary in their length of action in the body. This can increase the hazards of the drug. Many physicians and drug companies are urging parents to give their children long-acting preparations such as Concerta, Metadate ER, Ritalin SR, and Adderall XR. Some doctors and parents favor the long-acting preparations because they avoid the necessity of the child going to the school nursing office for an afternoon dose. Some physicians also hope that the longer-acting preparations will cause fewer emotional or behavioral ups and downs by maintaining a more consistent blood level.

However, when adverse reactions develop in response to a long-acting preparation, these reactions are likely to last longer after the drug is stopped. Anything from a severe headache or cardiac arrhythmia to a suicidal depression or a terrifying hallucination is likely to persist for many more hours due to the longer-lasting effect of the sustained-released preparations. Also keep in mind the danger described in Chapter 5—that longer-acting preparations are likely to be more neurotoxic. That is, they pose an even graver risk to the brain.

This concludes the overview of harmful effects caused by stimulant drugs. Keep in mind that even the "therapeutic effect" is really an adverse reaction—the crushing of spontaneous thought and behavior and the enforcement of obsessive thoughts and compulsive behaviors.

7

How Stimulants Cause Withdrawal, Addiction, and Abuse

The following remarkable warning appears in capital letters in a boxed section as the first item to be read in the Adderall and the Dexedrine labels:

AMPHETAMINES HAVE A HIGH POTENTIAL FOR ABUSE. ADMINISTRATION OF AMPHETAMINES FOR PROLONGED PERIODS OF TIME MAY LEAD TO DRUG DEPENDENCE AND MUST BE AVOIDED.[1]

Although it does not appear with the same strength in the Ritalin label, this statement is equally true for Ritalin and all of the other stimulants commonly used to treat children. It should also be taken as a warning that all of these drugs cause potentially severe withdrawal reactions.

Much of the medical profession acts as if it has never been admonished that stimulant administration for prolonged periods of time "must be avoided." Instead, long-term use of stimulants is often encouraged, and parents are told to keep their children on amphetamines for months and years.

If the medical profession were prescribing rationally, the fore-warning to avoid long-term administration, and the lack of evidence for any long-term efficacy, would utterly prevent the prescription of stimulants to children or adults for more than a few weeks' duration.

Withdrawal Reactions and Worsening Behavior

Symptoms of withdrawal can take place a few hours after the last dose of a stimulant, so that children commonly begin to go into withdrawal by the evening or the next morning. If a child's behavior appears to get worse or to deteriorate in any way a few hours or more after taking a stimulant drug, there's a high probability that the child is undergoing a withdrawal reaction.

Teachers often observe, "I can tell when Johnny hasn't taken his medication," meaning that they can see his behavior become more distressed or distressing. They don't realize that this is typically caused by a withdrawal reaction rather than by Johnny's own problems.

Parents and teachers sometimes believe that a child needs stimulants because the child's behavior deteriorates when one or two doses are missed. Such abrupt changes in a child are more likely due to withdrawal symptoms than to a child's inherent need for the drug. If we thought of alcohol or narcotics in the same way, we would think that alcoholics and narcotics addicts "needed" their drugs in order to be normal. In fact, they need to get free of their drugs in order to have a hope of becoming normal or healthy human beings.

The Ritalin label confirms, however inadequately, the danger of serious withdrawal problems. In a boxed section labeled "Drug Dependence," it states, "Careful supervision is required during drug withdrawal, since severe depression as well as the effects of chronic overactivity can be unmasked." The sentence is marred by spin doctoring that suggests that the symptoms are somehow being "unmasked" rather than directly caused by the Ritalin withdrawal. The label then states, "Long-term follow-up may be required because of the patient's basic personality disturbances." Again, this is spin doctoring of the fact that long-term exposure to these drugs, followed by withdrawal, can leave the patient with "basic personality disturbances" that the individual never had before taking stimulants.

The Meaning of Schedule II

Remember that Ritalin is an amphetamine-like drug that shares many characteristics with amphetamine, methamphetamine, and cocaine. Each of these drugs has been placed in Schedule II of all of the world's drug enforcement agencies to indicate that they are among the very most dangerous medications in regard to addiction and abuse.[2] Every stimulant mentioned in this book, with the exception of pemoline (Cylert), is in Schedule II. Ritalin, Ritalin SR, Ritalin LA, Focalin, Methylin, Concerta, Metadate ER, Dexedrine, DextroStat, Adderall, Adderall XR, and Desoxyn are all in Schedule II.

All of these stimulants are subject to diversion—that is, to abuse outside of their intended medical use. All of them are trafficked—that is, sold illegally in a systematic fashion.

At the consensus conference on ADHD and its treatment in 1998, an official representative of the U.S. Drug Enforcement Administration (DEA) issued a grave warning about the dangers of Ritalin as an addictive, abuse-prone drug:[3]

In summary, the DEA review shows that MPH [methylphenidate, or Ritalin] has a high abuse potential and is associated with a degree of diversion, abuse, and trafficking similar to that for other pharmaceutical Schedule II substances. Information from physicians, parents, schools, poison control centers, adolescent treatment centers, surveys, and law enforcement data suggested that a growing number of adolescents were using this drug illicitly, and that the primary source was individuals who have been prescribed this drug for ADHD, and that adolescents do not view abuse of this drug as serious. Physicians, parents, and school officials need to be alerted to take the necessary steps to safeguard against the diversion and abuse of this drug.

Another DEA publication asked the question, "How do Ritalin advocates respond to the mass of evidence concerning Ritalin addiction and abuse?" It answered, "Few, if any ADHD/Ritalin books for parents give proper emphasis to the drug's addictive capacities."[4]

Similarly, Sannerud and Feussner from the DEA's Office of Diversion Control (2000) recently reemphasized that animal experiments show that Ritalin has an "abuse liability similar to that of other Schedule II stimulants, including amphetamine, methamphetamine, and cocaine." Furthermore, they found that "data on abuse" in humans confirm that Ritalin "is diverted and abused to a similar extent as other pharmaceutical Schedule II substances."

The world's drug control agencies and addiction experts agree with the DEA that Ritalin and the amphetamine stimulants easily and frequently become abused and that Ritalin is similar to amphetamine and cocaine in its mental and addictive effects.[5] It is therefore shocking that so many drug advocates and ordinary physicians harbor a belief that these drugs do not present a danger for addiction and abuse.

Despite the claims of Novartis, the manufacturer of Ritalin, this drug is not a "mild" stimulant. In fact, Ritalin and all of the commonly used stimulants are very powerful, dangerous drugs, or they would not be placed in the Drug Enforcement Administration's Schedule II, indicating that they are the very most addictive and abuse-prone drugs used in medicine. Ritalin (methylphenidate) was in fact one of the very first drugs put into Schedule II when the classification system was established in the early 1970s.

Trying to Undermine the DEA

In 1994, the drug company Novartis attempted to make an end run around the DEA. CHADD, a parents' group that was at the time receiving large amounts of money from Novartis, lobbied the DEA to try to get it to drop Ritalin out of Schedule II.[6] This would have relieved Novartis of having to go to the DEA each year in order to get approval for the gross amount of Ritalin that it manufactures. It would have relieved doctors of the necessity of writing prescriptions, rather than calling them in, for Ritalin. It would have been a boon to Novartis and to organizations like CHADD that support the concept of ADHD and the use of stimulant drugs. Fortunately, the DEA fought back with scientific data on the dangers of Ritalin[7] and won. Ritalin remains in Schedule II. In *Talking Back to Ritalin* (rev. ed., 2001a) I have documented the details of the economics and politics of Ritalin and ADHD, including the partnership between CHADD and the drug company Novartis.

Creating Malfunctions in the Brain

The inclusion of all the commonly used stimulants in Schedule II not only tells us that they pose a high risk of addiction and withdrawal, it tells us that these drugs have a powerful impact on the brain. They cause addiction in part because they cause potentially painful and lasting withdrawal symptoms. When a child or adult takes these drugs, the function of the brain is distorted or impaired by the drug, so that when the drug is stopped, the brain persists in its abnormal function. Drug withdrawal symptoms are the result of this persistence of abnormal function after stopping the drug. Keep in mind, however, that the abnormalities of function take place while the child or adult is taking the stimulant; they merely become more obvious when the drug is abruptly withdrawn.

Addiction and abuse are complicated psychological and biological reactions. Drug abuse can be caused in part by direct drug effects, such as euphoria, that make people want to take them.

In routine prescription doses, stimulants don't usually cause euphoria. To achieve euphoria, the drugs are usually taken in larger doses or through very dangerous nasal or intravenous routes. Taken at ordinary doses, these drugs more often cause an emotional flatness or indifference that can provide a certain amount of relief from emotional suffering. They can also cause an artificial overfocusing that allows people to go on with anxiety-provoking or aggravating activities that they might otherwise want to avoid, such as studying, socializing, or public speaking. However, once the individual decides to stop taking the drug, the discomfort of withdrawal can play a major role in the continuing addiction to the drug.

Creating Future Cocaine Addicts

Studies have shown that normal animals can easily become addicted to methylphenidate and amphetamine. Waves of Ritalin addiction and abuse in various parts of the world during the 1960s led to its rapid inclusion in Schedule II of international drug enforcement agencies.

Animals addicted to cocaine will turn to Ritalin, amphetamine, or methamphetamine as a substitute for the cocaine. Similarly, human addicts are known to cross-addict to cocaine, Ritalin, and the amphetamines, depending on what's available at the moment. A variety of studies, including brain biochemistry and brain scans, have shown that all of the stimulants, including cocaine, have similar effects on the same chemical messengers and the same areas of the brain.

A very experienced team of experts who specialize in highly sophisticated studies of brain function published a lengthy report with the title "Is Methylphenidate Like Cocaine?"[8] This remarkable scientific document appeared in June 1995 in the American Medical Association publication the *Archives of General Psychiatry*. After reviewing many studies, the team concluded that Ritalin and cocaine have almost identical effects on the brain. The two drugs impact in a very similar fashion specific biochemical processes in the same regions of the brain and produce a similar "high" when given intravenously. The main difference is the more long-lasting effect of Ritalin. The authors speculated that the longer-lasting effect of Ritalin might make the drug less subject to abuse than cocaine. That is, by remaining active in the brain for a longer time, Ritalin might create a less drastic withdrawal and less dramatic need for repeated doses. Indeed, Ritalin tends to be less severely abused than cocaine, and its longer length of action may account for the difference.

In response to the article "Is Methylphenidate Like Cocaine?" an editorial was published in the same issue of the *Archives of General Psychiatry*.[9] The editorial concluded: "Cocaine, one of the most reinforcing and addictive of the abused drugs, has pharmacological actions very similar to those of MPH [Ritalin], one of the most commonly prescribed psychotropic medications for children in the United States."

What does all this mean in plain English? Ritalin's biochemical mechanism of action is essentially the same as that of cocaine, and therefore Ritalin produces similar effects to cocaine. In fact, all of the stimulants, including Ritalin and cocaine, jack up dopamine, serotonin, and norepinephrine chemical messengers in the brain, producing a variety of similar mental abnormalities. If given intravenously, the "high" is the same for all of them. When taken orally and in smaller doses, they have less of a punch than snorted and smoked cocaine; but they still have a punch and are strong enough to substitute for cocaine. Meanwhile, children will vary enormously in how they respond to a particular dose, but the long-term use of prescribed stimulants, even without achieving a high, can transform the brain into an organ that has become adjusted to stimulants and demands continuing stimulant use.

Because of the similarities among all the stimulants, including cocaine, it should have been no surprise when a recent study showed that children who are treated for ADHD with stimulants are more likely to abuse cocaine in young adulthood.[10] In my forensic work as a medical expert, I have evaluated cases in which prescribed stimulant use led to cocaine abuse in adolescence and in young adulthood. In two cases, the cocaine-abusing youngsters ended up killing someone.

Withdrawal Symptoms

Withdrawal symptoms are very common after even one dose of stimulant drugs. When withdrawal occurs soon after stopping the drug and involves a worsening of the individual's original symptoms, it is called "rebound." Scientific studies have shown that most children have rebound symptoms starting with their first dose of a stimulant. A study conducted at the National Institute of Mental Health found a dramatic degree of rebound after only one dose:[11]

> A marked behavioral rebound was observed by parents and teachers starting approximately 5 hours after medication had been given; this consisted of excitability, talkativeness, and, for three children, apparent euphoria.

Because they can occur within a few hours of the last dose of a stimulant, these withdrawal reactions can occur between doses of a drug. This is called "interdose withdrawal." It can lead to a child going through cycles of worsening behavior throughout the day and evening.

It is worth reemphasizing that parents and teachers often mistakenly decide that a child is benefiting from medication and needs medication after the child misses a dose and becomes more disturbed. In reality, a worsening of behavior following a missed dose of stimulant medication is much more likely to indicate a withdrawal reaction.

Often the withdrawal reaction is similar to the child's original problems but worse. To repeat, this is called "rebound." Even many doctors seem relatively unaware of these reactions. Like teachers and parents, they observe a withdrawal reaction and mistakenly conclude that the child benefits from and needs to be on medication. This misunderstanding about stimulant effects is one of the main reasons parents, teachers, and doctors decide that children should be continued on medication.

It is difficult to predict how an individual will react to withdrawal from stimulants. As the NIMH study demonstrated, very commonly children will undergo excitability. This can include insomnia, irritability, aggressiveness, and other signs of being "hyper." Withdrawal effects are often the opposite of the primary drug effect, and so children who have been flattened or subdued by the drug are likely to become more difficult than ever to manage during even brief interludes several hours after the last dose of the drug or when a dose is skipped.

Some children and adults who have been energized by taking stimulants are more likely to feel fatigued and severely unfocused during withdrawal. I have seen patients who have suffered from chronic, disabling exhaustion, as well as difficulty focusing, for months and even years after stopping the use of prescription stimulants such as Ritalin and Adderall.

Many children who take prescribed stimulants seem to be able to stop them with little or no difficulty. Any increased irritability and agitation, or crashing with fatigue, may last only a day or two. As a result, many parents take their children off the drugs during weekends and other breaks from school without encountering any serious problems. However, some children will undergo more severe withdrawal reactions when their parents try to stop the child's prescription stimulants. *In the extreme, the child may display psychotic symptoms or severe depression with suicidal impulses.* Chapter 8 will discuss how to safely withdraw from stimulant drugs.

In concluding, it is important to realize not only that stimulant addiction and abuse is a danger to the individual child or adult who takes the drug, but that the increasing use of stimulants poses a threat to all of society. First, as the DEA noted, the rampant prescription of such drugs to children has reinforced the false idea that these drugs are relatively harmless. This has encouraged other children and young adults to experiment with and to abuse them. Second, as the DEA has again warned, the widespread prescription of these drugs has made them easily available for diversion to illegal uses. Large batches have been stolen from school nursing offices. Young children have been showing up in emergency rooms with Ritalin toxicity from using the drug "recreationally." Some have died of heart attacks from snorting Ritalin.

I've already shown how the widespread use of stimulants to treat children diagnosed with ADHD is harming individual children and undermining the institutions of the family and school. It is also encouraging children to grow up under the influence of multiple psychiatric drugs and turning them into lifetime consumers for the psychopharmaceutical industry and psychiatry. Now we discover that it's also increasing drug addiction and abuse among our children and youth. The widespread use of psychoactive substances is simply not a good answer to our individual, family, or society problems and instead tends to worsen them.

8

How to Withdraw
from Stimulants

When withdrawing yourself, your children, or your patient from stimulant drugs, caution is the best approach. Overall, withdrawal from stimulant drugs can vary a great deal from person to person. Expect the unexpected and assume that almost anything that happens during withdrawal may be due to withdrawal.

In emergencies when an individual is suffering from a serious complication of a stimulant drug, such as cardiac arrhythmia, seizures, psychosis, tics or spasms, or a hypersensitivity reaction that interferes with breathing, it may be necessary to stop the medication immediately. When necessary, abrupt withdrawal can involve hospitalization for medical monitoring. But in the vast majority of cases, stimulant drug withdrawal can be done in a more regulated manner.

Especially when taking relatively small doses, such as the manufacturer's recommended starting doses, or when taking the medications for only a few weeks or months, many children and adults are able to stop the drugs abruptly with little or no harm. But even under these circumstances, some children will run into potentially serious difficulty when stopping the medication, especially during the first few days. A worsening of behavior is probably the most common withdrawal reaction. Among the more serious is "crashing," with the feeling of depression and even suicidal thoughts or actions. *Therefore, I always recommend that stimulants be withdrawn gradually with careful supervision.*

Principles of Stimulant Drug Withdrawal

There are several basic principles for the nonemergency withdrawal from any psychiatric medication:

First, go slowly enough to make it comfortable for the person undergoing the withdrawal. In this regard, there's no substitute for staying in close touch with what the person is feeling during the withdrawal period and for a sufficient time afterward.

Second, make sure that the child or adult has a good safety network of caring individuals who are aware that withdrawal is taking place. The child or adult undergoing withdrawal may be the last person to realize that a dangerous withdrawal reaction is occurring, especially if it is a mental reaction, such as depression or psychosis, that clouds judgment.

Third, if a person begins to experience an unacceptable level of discomfort or difficulty, it can usually be relieved by quickly returning to the previous dose. For example, if a child has been reduced from 40 mgs to 30 mgs of Ritalin per day before experiencing feelings of lethargy and depression, then a quick resumption of the 40 mg dose is likely to reverse the reaction. Then, after a suitable period of time and with great care, the withdrawal can be resumed, probably more slowly.

Fourth, if at all possible, find an experienced professional to help with the withdrawal, especially if the individual has been taking relatively large doses for a long period of time, and even more certainly if the individual is taking other drugs in addition to stimulants. Unfortunately, it can be very difficult to find knowledgeable health professionals willing to work with patients or their families to stop taking psychiatric drugs. It's commonplace to run into doctors who freely prescribe drugs after a few minutes in the office. But it's disappointingly difficult to find doctors who are as willing to help patients stop taking psychiatric medications.

If the original prescribing physician is unwilling to help you or your child withdraw from stimulants, you may find that your general practitioner or family doctor is willing to supervise the process. With coauthor David Cohen, I've written a book, *Your Drug May Be Your Problem: How and Why to Stop Taking Psychiatric Medications,* that can be useful to both the patient and the doctor. It's the only book published to date about withdrawing from psychiatric drugs with specific instructions relevant to every class of drug. Many professionals have found that book useful in developing their own guidelines to drug withdrawal, and you may want to provide your professional with *Your Drug May Be Your Problem* or with this book.

The guidelines in this book are intended to provide direction for withdrawing from stimulant drugs that have been taken in doses well within the range suggested by the manufacturer's label for the drug. If a person has been exposed to large doses or many months of medication, withdrawal can become a more serious problem. If other drugs are involved, withdrawal can become especially dangerous. If a child or adult is taking several psychiatric medications at once, withdrawal needs to be done with special care and under close supervision by an experienced professional. The suggested guidelines in this chapter cannot substitute for a professional consultation.

Especially if stimulants have been abused, hospitalization for withdrawal and a rehabilitation program may be required. Similarly, if serious psychiatric problems are present, additional treatment and especially careful supervision may be needed during the withdrawal process.

The Ten-Percent-per-Week Guideline

Clinicians often like to have a formula, even if it's a very rough one. That is, they want to have some idea about how fast or slow to go in withdrawing from drugs. If not interpreted too rigidly, the ten-percent-per-week guideline can be a helpful starting point to guide a clinician in withdrawing a patient from psychoactive drugs.

If you are concerned that a drug has been administered long enough to cause serious withdrawal reactions, a *minimum* ten weeks of withdrawal is a good rule of thumb. Using this guideline, you withdraw the person no more rapidly that one-tenth of the dose each week for ten weeks. At that point, there will be none remaining.

Ten weeks of gradual withdrawal will usually suffice to prevent any life-threatening consequences during withdrawal from almost any psychoactive or mind- and brain-altering drug. However, in difficult situations, withdrawal can take much longer than that. In regard to stimulants, though, it can usually be done more rapidly.

The ten-week guideline applies to withdrawing from one drug at a time. Withdrawing from two or more drugs can take much longer. It does not take into account the treatment of ongoing psychiatric problems.

In general, it's not good to impose a rigid schedule on yourself or anyone else when it comes to withdrawing from addictive substances such as nicotine, alcohol, opiates, sedative tranquilizers, or stimulant medications. If at all possible, the patient shouldn't go any faster than he or she can comfortably tolerate.

A Positive Outcome from Helping Your Child Withdraw from Stimulants

If you are going to help your child withdraw from stimulants, you need to be in very close touch with your child and all of your child's caregivers, including clinicians, teachers, and babysitters, during the withdrawal period. Your child and his or her teachers should know how to get a hold of you during school hours. The babysitter should be able to locate you when you're out of the house. You should personally be checking with your child in the morning, afternoon, and evening to find out how he or she is feeling and behaving. You should tuck your child into bed at night and welcome your child into the world in the morning.

If you do all of these things during the withdrawal period, you may find that you like relating this way to your child. It's actually a healthy approach to normal parenting. Through making withdrawal safe and then applying the approach to everyday life, you may end up improving your relationship with your child and making your child's life more safe and secure overall.

The Physical Basis of Withdrawal

The physical basis of withdrawal was touched upon in discussing rebound and other withdrawal phenomena in earlier chapters. When the brain has been exposed to any psychoactive agent, it attempts to counteract its effects. That is, the brain attempts to overcome the drug effect. As a result, during withdrawal the individual is likely to experience the opposite of the drug effect.

If smoking cigarettes tends to "calm your nerves," then abruptly stopping cigarettes is likely to leave you with very jangled nerves. Similarly, if you take sedatives or drink alcohol in order to fall asleep more easily, after a while your brain will become hyperactive in an attempt to keep you awake despite the pills or alcohol. Abruptly stopping the sleeping aids is then likely to leave you in a state of worsened insomnia.

The same thing happens to the brain when it is exposed to stimulants. The brain fights back. Once again, the most common withdrawal effects from stimulants are the opposite of the drug's effects. However, particularly in regard to stimulants, withdrawal effects can take many different forms.

If the drugs have suppressed a child's spontaneous behavior, then you can expect the behavior to worsen during the withdrawal period. This is very common and can even happen toward the end of the day, when the effect of the morning or early afternoon dose is wearing off.

Although their behavior may be suppressed, some children also become "wired" or anxious and agitated on Ritalin. During withdrawal, they may collapse into a state of apathy and exhaustion and sleep a great deal. A child who has lost his or her appetite on the drug may become voraciously hungry for a while.

A Personal Experience

I had an experience that informed me more personally about the potential impact of stimulant withdrawal.

Caffeine is a very mild stimulant compared to Ritalin, Focalin, Adderall, and other stimulants used to treat ADHD. At a time when I was working under some high-pressure book deadlines, I got into the habit of drinking three or four mugs of coffee each day. I was unaware that the coffee was having much of an effect on me, but I nonetheless felt like I "needed it."

Then one afternoon I unexpectedly became very tired and grumpy. Although I rarely napped in the afternoon, I felt like going to sleep on the couch instead of working. I thought I might be getting the flu. I had developed a wicked headache, making me think it was a virulent virus. I also felt as if something were the matter with me emotionally, almost as if I were getting a little sad or depressed. Being a psychiatrist, I naturally began to think about all the things that might be upsetting me, but nothing in particular came to mind. I felt like I needed more coffee, so I drank a couple of extra mugs, to no avail.

That night I slept like the dead. In the morning I felt somewhat less exhausted and the headache was mostly gone, but I was definitely foggy in the head. It was as if the gears were grinding in my brain rather than running smoothly. By midmorning I continued to improve, but I still didn't feel like myself.

At that point, my wife Ginger came to me looking very sheepish and apologetic. She knew what was the matter with me. The day before, she had accidentally filled the coffee can with decaffeinated coffee. I was going through caffeine withdrawal.

Keep in mind that caffeine is a relatively mild stimulant with relatively mild withdrawal effects. Now imagine that a child is being withdrawn from a strong stimulant, such as Ritalin, Concerta, or Adderall, and that the child was already experiencing emotional difficulties even before the withdrawal began. It's easy to see how a child's mental condition and behavior could worsen and even deteriorate during withdrawal from stimulants.

Permanent Withdrawal Symptoms

I have evaluated and treated adults who have had very serious problems withdrawing from prolonged exposure to high doses of stimulants prescribed by physicians. Some have continued to experience withdrawal symptoms for an indefinite period of time years after stopping the drug. They have suffered from chronic fatigue, restlessness, and difficulty focusing their attention. Some have had memory impairment and difficulty thinking as clearly or effectively as in the past. In medical terms, they suffer from generalized cognitive deficits.

These individuals are suffering from permanent changes in the brain caused by a combination of direct toxic effects and compensatory brain changes. Thus, part of the irreversible problem is due to harmful effects from direct exposure and part to the brain's reactions to the drugs.

These people were not obtaining the stimulants illegally. Doctors had been prescribing them, albeit sometimes in too large doses with too little supervision of the patient and sometimes with no real justification. Individuals who abuse stimulants and obtain them illegally are also likely to develop long-term or even permanent mental impairments.

Despite the potential risks, most children and adults stop taking prescribed stimulants without a great deal of difficulty, especially if they've taken them in relatively small doses for a relatively short period of time. If you are accustomed to taking your child off stimulant medication on weekends, holidays, or summer vacation, then you already have some experience with how your child reacts to abrupt withdrawal. Usually the worst of the withdrawal is over in a few days, so if your child has previously easily gotten through two- or three-day weekends or holidays without the medication, there is a good likelihood that nothing more serious will turn up after the third or fourth day.

After the first few days of successfully stopping the stimulant medication for your child, the potentially most difficult challenges will begin. First, you will have to address the reasons that you originally put your child on the drug.

Second, if taken for many months or years, the stimulant drug will have delayed your child's mental and emotional growth and development, adding new problems to the ones that already existed. Having dispensed with the drug, you will need to find the necessary human resources in yourself and your child's teachers and other caregivers.

Third, when children are told that they have "ADHD" and need medications to control their behavior, they are in effect taught not to believe in their own ability to control themselves. Your child will need reeducation in what it means to exert self-control and self-discipline. At the same time, as a parent or teacher, your belief in ADHD and drugs has undermined your confidence that your child or student can be reached through improved parenting or teaching. You will have to reempower yourself to help your child or student mature. You may find it necessary, and fulfilling, to spend much more time than in the past with your child.

The concluding chapters of the book will make some practical suggestions toward reempowering yourself and the children in your care.

Do Stimulants Really Help with "ADHD"?

Pronouncements made in public by professional advocates for stimulants paint glowing pictures about the effectiveness of these drugs. But professional reviews and textbooks often present a much more conservative picture—one that hardly justifies exposing children to such grave dangers.

A review in the American Psychiatric Press *Textbook of Psychiatry* concluded:

> Stimulants do not produce lasting improvements in aggressivity, conduct disorder, criminality, education achievement, job functioning, marital relationships, or long-term adjustment.[1]

Similarly, one NIMH study concluded that "the long-term efficacy of stimulant medication has not been demonstrated in *any* domain of child function,"[2] and another by respected researchers confirmed there is no "long-term advantage" to taking stimulants.[3]

A very thorough review sponsored by the U.S. Department of Education came to conclusions that would startle most people

who have been exposed to pro-drug advocacy.[4] The following is
taken verbatim from the report:

> Long-term beneficial effects have not been verified by re-
> search.
> Stimulant medication may improve learning in some
> cases but impair learning in others.
> Teachers and parents should not expect significantly im-
> proved reading or athletic skills, positive social skills, or
> learning of new concepts.
> Teachers and parents should not expect long-term im-
> provement in academic achievement or reduced antiso-
> cial behavior.

There is no doubt that in the short term, stimulant drugs can
suppress the behavior of children and make them temporarily
easier to manage and be around, and in some cases make it easier to compel them to carry out rote, boring tasks. But the drugs
do nothing else for the child, while exposing the youngster to
considerable harm.

Despite decades of research attempts, no evidence has been developed to show that stimulants improve a child's learning, academic achievement, psychological or mental state, social relationships, or overall future. In reality, stimulants do nothing but
suppress the child's overall spontaneity while enforcing obsessive-compulsive behaviors.

What about the long term? When all of the stimulant labels and
most of the textbooks admit that there's no evidence for anything
but a short-term effect, what do they mean by "short term"?

The Meaning of "Short Term" and "Long Term"

In regard to the most recently approved stimulant drug, Adderall
XR, only two controlled clinical trials were required for approval,
and those two trials lasted for a mere three weeks. Under the sub-
heading "Long-Term Use," the label itself states that "the effec-

tiveness of ADDERALL XR™ for long-term use, i.e., *for more than 3 weeks*, has not been systematically evaluated in controlled clinical trials."[5] The Adderall XR label admits that there is no evidence for the drug's safety or efficacy beyond these three weeks.

Adderall XR is a new long-acting preparation of the same amphetamine mixture found in the original Adderall preparation. For how long was the original Adderall tested? The label for Adderall repeats the statement that "long-term effects of amphetamines in children have not been well-established," but it doesn't tell us how long Adderall was tested for. In fact, the label for Adderall provides no controlled clinical trial data at all! It is one of the most skimpy drug labels approved in psychiatry in recent years.

Notice that the FDA-approved Adderall label makes a blanket statement in regard to all amphetamines—that none of them have been adequately studied long-term in regard to their effects on children (or adults). But for how long have amphetamines been approved for use in controlling the behavior of children? For nearly fifty years! In all that time, despite many attempts, long-term safety and efficacy (i.e., beyond a few weeks) has not been established.

One stimulant drug label after another has been "grandfathered" into place by permitting the use of very old and useless data. As Chapter 12 will document, the basic information on adverse reactions for Ritalin, Ritalin SR, Dexedrine, Adderall, and Adderall XR can be traced back to labels that were already outdated in 1973–1974. To a great extent, the same is true in regard to efficacy studies. The FDA accepts the efficacy claims for stimulants based on original studies for FDA approval that were conducted in the 1950s for Ritalin and Dexedrine. Needless to say, studies in 1950s were grossly inadequate by today's standards, FDA monitoring was negligible at that time, and the drug companies heavily manipulated the data.

In recent years, many short-term studies, usually four to six weeks in duration, have confirmed that stimulants do indeed have an effect on many children for that brief period of time. But the effect is always the same: that basic overall suppression of behavior and enforcement of attention to rote tasks.

Something Fishy?

If the most recently approved stimulant medication has only been tested for three weeks in controlled clinical trials, does this smell like something fishy is going on? If most studies over many decades have lasted only a mere four to six weeks, does that also sound suspicious?

There are two possible reasons that clinical trials for stimulants are limited to only a few weeks at a time.

First, the drugs do not work long-term, so the trials have to be short in order to look good.

Second, the drugs are so hazardous that most children cannot be made to stay on them for more than a few weeks.

There is evidence that both of these forces are at work. Long-term efficacy has remained unproven after almost fifty years because the drugs don't work after a few weeks and because they are too hazardous for sufficient numbers of patients to stay on for more than a few weeks at a time.

One of the very few longer-term studies was published in 1997 amid a great deal of media fanfare.[6] It lasted fifteen months and claimed to show a positive effect. However, ten of the original seventy-two children (14 percent) dropped out within one month due to a combination of no drug effect and adverse effects; and of the original participants, approximately one-third completed the study. For these and other reasons, the study has been largely discredited and is seldom mentioned.

A Government Hoax

NIMH gathered together a group of dedicated stimulant advocates and funded them at six separate locations to conduct long-term research on stimulant drugs. The avowed purpose was to end the ADHD/stimulant controversy on a favorable note for the drugs.

When the fourteen-month-long study (MTA Cooperative Group, 1999a, 1999b) was finally published, I was so dismayed that I devoted an entire chapter to it in *Talking Back to Ritalin* (rev. ed., 2001a) and published a critical analysis in professional journals.[7]

Basically, the NIMH project failed to meet the two most basic criteria for a scientific study. First, it had no placebo (sugar pill) control group. Therefore, there was no way to tell whether the changes in the children would or would not have occurred if the drugs had never been given. Second, there were no double-blind evaluators. Everyone from parents and teachers to doctors knew which children were taking the drugs, so the strong investigator bias in favor of the drug could run rampant. In addition, the only "blind" evaluators were in the classroom, and they found no positive drug effect.

From a scientific viewpoint, the study was worthless. What it really reveals is the desperation of its organizers, including psychiatrist Peter Jensen, to justify the ongoing epidemic of child drugging. Meanwhile, the most avid drug advocates continue to fail to provide evidence for any positive long-term effects for stimulants. And long-term means beyond a few weeks of suppressed behavior!

Massive Overdrugging Even by Official Standards

If doctors and other advocates of ADHD and stimulants paid attention to existing professional standards for prescribing stimulants, far fewer children would be taking these drugs.

The 2001 Ritalin label instructs the prescribing physician:

> Stimulants are not intended for use in the child who exhibits symptoms secondary to environmental factors and/or primary psychiatric disorders, including psychosis. Appropriate educational placement is essential and psychosocial intervention is generally necessary. When remedial measures alone are insufficient, the decision to prescribe stimulant medication will depend upon the physician's assessment of the chronicity and severity of the child's symptoms.

The Ritalin label also instructs the prescribing physician:

Prescription should not depend solely on the presence of one or more of the behavioral characteristics. When these symptoms are associated with acute stress reactions, treatment with Ritalin is not usually indicated. Long-term effects of Ritalin in children have not been well established.

Similar observations can be found in other stimulant labels. It is instructive to review the principles and practices that can be summarized from these pithy paragraphs that pertain not only to Ritalin but to all stimulants:

1. *Stimulant prescription should not depend solely on the child meeting the official diagnostic criteria for ADHD.*

In real life, parents and patients are given the idea that the mere diagnosis of ADHD warrants the use of medication.

2. *Stimulants should not be prescribed if the behaviors are caused by environmental problems.*

The vast majority of children with ADHD-like symptoms are in fact suffering from environmental stressors in the school or home, and many do better as soon as they change teachers or schools, as soon as school is over for the summer, or as soon as their families learn better child-rearing principles and practices.

3. *Stimulants should not be prescribed if the child is primarily suffering from another psychiatric disorder, such as psychosis, stress reactions, anxiety, obsessive-compulsive problems, post-traumatic stress disorder, adjustment reactions, depression, and so on.*

Yet doctors too often prescribe Ritalin for behaviors that are driven by anxiety, stress, or other psychosocial problems.

4. *Educational, remedial, and psychosocial interventions are usually necessary. That is, efforts need to be made to improve the school and family life of the child.*

Too many prescribing doctors pay no attention whatsoever to these requirements and instead prescribe stimulants without taking the time to look into more helpful interventions in the school and home.

5. *When remedial interventions themselves are insufficient, then the doctor can consider medication.*

Giving medications should not be automatic. Even when psychosocial interventions haven't worked, doctors can "consider" medication without necessarily prescribing it. Yet too many doctors prescribe before finding out if remedial interventions have been sufficient.

6. *Long-term effects of stimulants in children "have not been well established."*

This statement remains on all stimulant labels to this very day.

In addition, the official ADHD diagnosis as defined in the American Psychiatric Association's *Diagnostic and Statistical Manual of Mental Disorders* (1994, 2000) requires that the child was impaired by symptoms before age 7 and that the impairment occurs in two or more settings. Once again, doctors too often ignore these requirements when making the diagnosis and prescribing stimulants.

In making these criticisms, I do not want to imply that our children would be adequately served if the medical profession adhered to more accurate diagnosing and more stringent guidelines for the prescription of medication. The health professions would best serve the needs of our children by discarding the ADHD diagnosis and rejecting the use of medication to control their behavior.

We are exposing millions of children to dangerous stimulant drugs that have no proven effect beyond a few weeks and whose actual impact involves suppressing the brain and mental function. The use of these drugs should be abandoned in favor of meeting the real needs of our children in the school and family.

Do Antidepressants and Other Drugs Help with "ADHD"?

Psychiatric drug treatment tends to run in fads. At the present moment, several fads in the treatment of children have converged in a most dangerous fashion:

- Using stimulants and other drugs as the first and only approach to treating children who have correctable environmental problems such as inadequate teaching at school or poor discipline at home.
- Prescribing multiple psychiatric drugs at once.
- Treating children with drugs that are not FDA-approved for anyone under age eighteen.
- Treating "ADHD" or behavior problems with especially dangerous antipsychotic or neuroleptic drugs intended for adults diagnosed with schizophrenia or psychosis.
- Treating the adverse effects of stimulants and antidepressants, such as tics and psychoses, by prescribing even more hazardous neuroleptics.
- Prescribing antidepressants such as Prozac, Paxil, Zoloft, Celexa, Luvox, and Effexor that commonly cause severe adverse drug reactions in children, including mania and psychosis.

- Diagnosing children with bipolar (manic-depressive) disorder, obsessive-compulsive disorder, and other psychiatric problems when they are in fact suffering from stimulant-induced and antidepressant-induced emotional disturbances.

It's no mystery how these trends get started. Drug companies hire "consultants" to preach their wares to the unwary doctor. Often without identifying the drug company as their patron, these doctors make unsubstantiated claims in seminars and journals for using these drugs for the treatment of children. The mystery to me is how so many practicing physicians can be hoodwinked into such dangerous practices.

Children diagnosed with ADHD are likely to be started on stimulant medication, but they frequently end up taking one or more additional psychiatric drugs. Much as happened to Alec (Chapter 2), doctors will often prescribe other drugs in order to handle the stimulant's adverse effects, such as insomnia, anxiety, agitation, obsessions and compulsions, or depression. Some children will develop psychotic symptoms on stimulants, including paranoid feelings, manic or "high" reactions, delusions, and visual, auditory, or tactile hallucinations. After the child begins to take two or more drugs that affect the brain and mind, he or she becomes an experiment in which almost any adverse mental effect can develop, as well as untold physical ones.

Starting with the first dose, almost any psychiatric drug, from the stimulants to the antidepressants, can worsen the symptoms commonly thought of as ADHD-like, especially difficulties with cognition and loss of self-control. Cognitive processes such as attention, memory, and learning are among the first functions to be impaired by the persistent use of almost any psychoactive drug including stimulants like Ritalin and cocaine and sedatives like Klonopin and alcohol.

People who persistently use psychoactive drugs legally or illegally for several months or more are likely to become forgetful, overlook details, and lose their focus on difficult tasks. Similarly, they may begin to experience "disinhibition" or "loss of impulse control." The earliest signs are irritability and unexpected outbursts of anger, followed eventually by dangerous expressions of violence. I have seen this pattern evolve in dozens of clinical and legal cases involving both children and adults.

Prozac-Like Antidepressants

This section summarizes material I have documented in enormous detail in several other books,[1] including an up-to-date chapter on children in *The Antidepressant Fact Book* (2001b).

Prozac-like antidepressants include Prozac (fluoxetine), Zoloft (sertraline), Paxil (paroxetine), Celexa (citalopram), and Luvox (fluvoxamine). These drugs block the removal of a neurotransmitter—serotonin—from its active place in the synapses between neurons in the brain.[2] Other antidepressants, including Effexor (venlafaxine), can do the same thing, but less selectively.

No antidepressants are approved for the treatment of depression in children because they don't work and because they cause mental and physical problems in children. Recently, while investigating a drug company's files in a legal case, I came across a letter from the FDA telling the drug company to stop trying to get their adult antidepressant approved for children. The FDA reminded the company that antidepressants don't work and have increased adverse effects in children.

Psychiatric drug prescription to children is too often driven by something other than science. Frequently it is motivated by the desire to prescribe drugs on the part of physicians who literally don't know any other approach to treating children. As a result, increasing numbers of children are being prescribed Prozac-like antidepressants.

All of the antidepressants in use today, including the Prozac-like drugs, can cause stimulation very similar to that caused by Ritalin and amphetamines such as Adderall and Dexedrine. Much like with the stimulants, there is a continuum of stimulation with insomnia and feeling "hyper" at the level of least intensity, and then increasing degrees of anxiety and agitation with the potential for manic and psychotic reactions. However, antidepressants produce paradoxical effects more frequently than the stimulants, sometimes resulting in sedation and increased sleep.

Drug-induced mania is a very dangerous disorder that can result in extreme and even outrageous and violent behavior. How often do children and young people on antidepressants become manic? Very, very often! In one controlled clinical trial of Prozac in depressed children, 6 percent had to drop out because of manic symptoms.[3] The label for Luvox in the *Physicians' Desk Reference* cites a rate of 4 percent for mania in children during similar clinical trials. These are extraordinarily high rates and should be sufficient to stop physicians from prescribing these and similar antidepressants to children.

Unfortunately, the real rates for antidepressant-induced mania as found in routine clinical practice are likely to be even higher. In clinical practice compared to research trials, the drugs are given for more than a few weeks, often in combination with other drugs, and with much less strict supervision. Consistent with this, a retrospective examination of hospital charts at the University of Pittsburgh found that 23 percent of youngsters treated with Prozac developed manic symptoms or mania.[4] Once again, such high rates of mania in themselves should stop the prescription of these drugs to children.

Even without becoming manic, children taking Prozac-like drugs often develop disturbed and aggressive behavior. A study of children in both clinical trials and routine clinic treatment at Yale University found that six out of forty-two (14 percent) developed suicidal or violent impulses on Prozac. A twelve-year-old boy taking Prozac suffered from such powerful nightmares about committing a school shooting that he began to lose track of reality and had to be hospitalized. Fortunately, the impulses went away when the Prozac was stopped. This was not a copycat nightmare since it took place before the rash of actual school shootings. Several years later, Eric Harris, one of the two school shooters at Columbine High School in Colorado, was taking Luvox when he committed the worst school shootings in American history.[5]

Antidepressants, like stimulants, commonly cause depression. While this may seem "paradoxical" and unexpected, it is reported time and again in studies for FDA approval of the newer antidepressants. Looking within the then-secret files of Eli Lilly and Company, the manufacturer of Prozac, I found that depressed patients made suicide attempts several times more frequently on Prozac than on placebo (sugar pill) or on older antidepressants. Since the Prozac, the placebo, and the older drugs were being given to the same or similar patients, it must be concluded that Prozac was the cause of the increased suicide-attempt rate. One of the drug company's own consultants suggested that the increased suicide-attempt rate could be due to Prozac's tendency to be stimulating. Meanwhile, the drug company, Eli Lilly, continues to keep this vital data under wraps as if it did not exist.

Lobotomy-Like Effects Caused by SSRIs

Closely related to the tendency for selective serotonin reuptake inhibitors to cause depression, they also cause a lobotomy-like indifference in children and adults. I may have been the first to warn about how SSRIs cause individuals to become relatively emotionless, and to lose their interest in themselves and their loved ones. The phenomenon has now become sufficiently accepted to be included in textbooks. The 1999 edition of the American Psychiatric Press *Textbook of Psychiatry*[6] devotes a section to "Apathy Syndromes" caused by SSRIs and compares the adverse drug effect to a "frontal lobe syndrome," that is, the flatness and lack of caring displayed by patients who have been surgically lobotomized with destruction of frontal-lobe tissue and function.

The American Psychiatric Press textbook warns that the drug-induced syndrome can be mistaken for a relapse into depression.

This, of course, could result in an increase in medication and a continued worsening of the individual's condition. This is one way in which children end up on increasing amounts and even numbers of antidepressants while they continue to get more apathetic and depressed, as well as emotionally and behaviorally out of control.

A report in 2001 in the *Journal of Child and Adolescent Psychopharmacology* describes five children who developed an SSRI-induced lobotomy syndrome, which the authors call an "Amotivational syndrome," that is, a mental condition characterized by lack of motivation.[7] They were taking Prozac or Paxil in low to moderate doses.

Since it took several weeks for the adverse effect to become apparent, its connection to the antidepressant drug was easily missed. In addition, children and teenagers often go through periods in which they seem "not to care" about school and family activities, adding to the tendency to overlook a direct connection to the drug.

One of the children also developed "disinhibition," with behavior that insulted and alienated adults and peers alike. I have evaluated the cases of teenagers and young adults who developed SSRI-induced apathy syndromes that eventually turned into violence.

The lack of motivation had other serious consequences. A seventeen-year-old girl's drug-induced lack of participation in her athletics had a "lasting impact on her career plans" and she did not go to college.

The children sometimes did not recognize that they had become apathetic. At other times, the youngsters, or their parents, preferred the reduction in anxiety that accompanied the overall reduction in the capacity to feel. From my perspective, this is a self-defeating viewpoint. When parents and children participate in family-oriented psychotherapy, the child's anxiety problems can often be overcome. Sometimes they are simply outgrown. Meanwhile, a drug-induced lack of motivation or caring will impair learning and psychosocial maturation, retarding the individual's overall development.

While children and adults seem to recover from these apathy syndromes when the drug is reduced or stopped, SSRIs are known to produce lasting changes in brain chemistry. This should sound an alarm about the potential for producing irreversible lobotomy syndromes. However, it is unlikely that any drug company will conduct the kind of long-term and potentially self-incriminating studies required to test for these tragic outcomes. Nor is the FDA likely to alienate the politically influential drug companies by requiring these studies.

The lobotomy-like syndrome caused by SSRIs is one more reason never to give these drugs to children and youth.

Causing Permanent Brain Damage

SSRI antidepressants not only cause serious emotional and behavioral disturbances in children, they also cause neurological problems that indicate underlying brain dysfunction. For example, they cause permanent tics and spasms somewhat similar to the tardive dyskinesia reaction experienced by Alec (Chapter 2; see "Antipsychotic Drugs" in the next section).

Very little research has been done on antidepressants to determine whether they cause permanent damage to the brain, but I have written extensively in my books about why we should anticipate this danger, especially in children. Remember that shrinkage in the brain has turned up in multiple studies of children taking stimulants and that it has been falsely attributed to "ADHD." Now brain damage is showing up in the brains of young animals on Prozac and children on Paxil.[8]

Even though some of the antidepressants are FDA approved for other purposes in children, such as obsessive-compulsive disorder, the newer antidepressants in particular are too dangerous to give to children.

The older antidepressants called tricyclics are also very dangerous for children to take. These drugs include imipramine, desipramine (Norpramin), nortriptyline (Pamelor, Aventyl), amitriptyline (Elavil), clomipramine (Anafranil), and doxepin

(Sinequan). In particular, they can cause potentially fatal cardiac arrhythmias. Children taking them should have regular physical examinations, blood tests, and electrocardiograms.

Antipsychotic or Neuroleptic Drugs

Doctors prescribing for children in a rational manner should avoid using neuroleptic (antipsychotic) drugs, given their enormous risks and their lack of demonstrated effectiveness. But in recent times, parents have regularly consulted me after these drugs have been prescribed to their children. In many cases, the children have been permanently damaged. They will live the remainder of their lives afflicted with drug-induced tardive dyskinesia, a disorder involving disfiguring and sometimes painful and disabling tics and spasms of the muscles.

Because doctors sometimes fail in their duty to tell parents about the nature of these drugs, I will list them:

The *older antipsychotic or neuroleptic drugs* include Haldol (haloperidol), Orap (pimozide), Mellaril (thioridazine), Prolixin (fluphenazine), Thorazine (chlorpromazine), Trilafon (perphenazine), Moban (molindone), Stelazine (trifluoperazine), Loxitane (loxapine), Serentil (mesoridazine), and Navane (thiothixene). Although sometimes promoted as a new drug, Clozaril (clozapine) is another old neuroleptic drug, one that was banned years ago in some European countries. Asendin (amoxapine) is marketed as an antidepressant but is in fact a neuroleptic, with all the dangers associated with these drugs. Etrafon and Triavil combine an antidepressant (amitriptyline) with a neuroleptic (perphenazine) and therefore share all the dangers of the neuroleptics.

The *newer antipsychotic or neuroleptic drugs* include Risperdal (risperidone), Zyprexa (olanzapine), Seroquel (quetiapine), and Geodon (ziprasidone).

In addition, several neuroleptic drugs are prescribed to children for gastrointestinal (GI) problems, such as gastric reflux, nausea, and vomiting. These drugs include Reglan (metoclopramide) and Compazine (prochlorperazine). Another drug, Propulsid (cisapride), was widely used to treat gastric problems in children until it was recently taken off the market. It has neuroleptic activity and causes the adverse effects associated with neuroleptic drugs.

An antihistamine, Phenergan (promethazine), is also used to treat various illnesses in children and has relatively weak neuroleptic activity that can, in some cases, cause or contribute to neuroleptic-induced neurological disorders. I am a consultant in a number of cases of severe, irreversible neurological disorders caused by the use of all of these drugs used for treating gastric reflux and related GI problems in children.

Two Adverse Reactions to Neuroleptics

Antipsychotic or neuroleptic drugs cause so many adverse effects that it would take a book to fully review them.[9] Two particular neurological effects of these drugs are remarkably common and potentially devastating, yet are readily overlooked by doctors. The two reactions are neuroleptic malignant syndrome and tardive dyskinesia.

Advocates for the antipsychotics will sometimes claim that one or another particular drug, especially newer ones, present a less frequent risk for causing these two dread disorders. However, the FDA requires every antipsychotic drug, including the newer ones like Risperdal, Zyprexa, Seroquel, and Geodon, to carry specific warnings about neuroleptic malignant syndrome and tardive dyskinesia.

Neuroleptic malignant syndrome can occur at any time, starting with the first dose. It acts very much like a viral inflammation of the brain (encephalitis) with mental disturbances increasing to possible coma and death. It usually includes fever, cardiovascular problems, and severe abnormal movements. It can occur in varying degrees and is often mistaken for an infection or even for a mental disorder. Many doctors seem to believe that neuroleptic malignant syndrome is rare, but actual studies show that it is common. A retrospective review of medical charts disclosed a rate of 2.4 percent—an extremely high rate for such a devastating disorder.[10]

Tardive dyskinesia was discussed in Chapter 2 in regard to the twitches and spasms of Alec's face and jaw. Tardive dyskinesia involves abnormal movements that are highly variable and can afflict any muscle of the body that is under voluntary control, including the face, eyes, tongue, neck, arms and legs, and torso. Breathing, speech, and swallowing can be impaired. In children, tardive dyskinesia often involves larger muscle groups such as the neck and shoulders or the torso, causing gross impairments, including difficulty standing or walking. This drug-induced disorder is usually irreversible, and there is no effective treatment.

Astronomical Rates of Tardive Dyskinesia

Rates for neuroleptic-induced tardive dyskinesia are astronomical. The most conservative (pro-drug) sources cite a rate of 3–5 percent cumulative per year.[11] According to this estimate, anyone taking these drugs would face a risk of at least 15–25 percent over five years. Rates in children are not so clearly established, but as I first emphasized in my 1983 medical book, the rates seem to be at least as high in children as in adults and the results are often more devastating, frequently involving severe mental disturbances and more disabling abnormal movements.

Variations of Tardive Dyskinesia

I have evaluated children who have been mistakenly diagnosed as suffering from epileptic "seizures" when their eyes rolled back in their head and their necks and backs arched in pain during muscle spasms caused by tardive dyskinesia. When painful muscle spasms are involved, this form of tardive dyskinesia is called tardive dystonia. Other children may suffer from an agitation with hyperactivity, so that they cannot sit or stand still. They are driven into repeated episodes of constant motion. The experience is like being tortured from inside their own body. This form of tardive dyskinesia is called tardive akathisia.

Overall, tardive dyskinesia can present itself in so many seemingly bizarre manifestations that uninformed physicians may be baffled by what is occurring. Also, tardive dyskinesia can wax and wane for no apparent reason, it can sometimes be partially controlled with great effort, it tends to worsen with stress or tiredness, and it usually disappears during sleep. These factors can also make the diagnosis confusing, especially to physicians who lack sufficient knowledge about the nature of the disorder. Some cases initially go undiagnosed or are blamed on the child's "mental illness" or "hyperactivity." As a result, the offending drugs are continued or even increased in dose, ultimately causing the development of a very severe case.

Prescribing physicians should carefully warn and educate parents about the dangers of these drugs and should regularly and thoroughly examine any child who is taking them. If at all possible, the physician should stop all neuroleptic or antipsychotic drugs at the first sign or hint of any kind of abnormal movement that could possibly be related to tardive dyskinesia. Because the drugs "mask," or cover up, the very symptoms they are creating, it is important to stop the drugs in order to do a proper assessment. On my web site, www.breggin.com, I have described some of the guidelines for treating patients with tardive dyskinesia and a number of cases in which I have been a medical consultant.

Risperdal, Too Often an Unrecognized Danger

Risperdal (risperidone) at present seems to be one of the neuroleptics mostly commonly prescribed in a negligent fashion to children with ADHD and behavior problems. The FDA has not approved its use for ADHD or for children. I am a medical consultant in many malpractice suits in which children have been damaged by this drug, including permanent disfigurement of the eyes and face in young children. Often, Risperdal is given after other drugs such as stimulants have worsened the child's behavior.

Too many doctors have received the mistaken idea that Risperdal is somehow safer than other neuroleptics in regard to causing tardive dyskinesia when it is in fact no better, and perhaps worse, than Haldol, a drug with a documented high rate of causing tardive dyskinesia.[12]

Causing Instead of Curing Tics and Tourette's Disorder

Because these drugs can temporarily mask or suppress tardive dyskinesia, as well as tics and spasms from other causes, they are sometimes used to treat tics and spasms. I have seen unscrupulous doctors attempt to hide tardive dyskinesia by increasing the doses of the neuroleptic while telling the patient or parents, "There's nothing to worry about." For a time, the abnormal movements seem to disappear, only to break through again with a more devastating severity.

Haldol and Orap are neuroleptics that are FDA approved for the control of Tourette's disorder, a combination of tics and compulsive vocalizations, such as making sounds or uttering inappropriate words. It seems incomprehensible that the FDA would approve drugs for the treatment of Tourette's when the same drugs are known to cause a very high rate of even more severe irreversible tics and spasms.

When a child develops tics or spasms as a result of taking stimulants such as Ritalin or Adderall, some doctors have been known to prescribe neuroleptics to temporarily mask or suppress the symptoms. The end result can be tragic and can take the form of even more severe, painful, disfiguring, and disabling abnormal movements.

Blaming Mothers for Poisoning Their Children

Because these neuroleptic drugs produce such a seemingly bizarre array of symptoms, some doctors have failed to recognize the harmful effects of their drugs and have instead falsely blamed parents for "poisoning" their own infants and children. These doctors have accused the parents, usually the mother, of suffering from Munchausen's by Proxy, a psychiatric disorder in which one person makes another person sick in other to receive attention and support from health professionals.

I have evaluated cases in which parents have been falsely accused of poisoning their children or otherwise causing them harm. In these cases, their infants or children developed gastric reflux or other GI problems and were negligently treated with drugs like Reglan, Propulsid, Compazine, and Phenergan. Especially in the case of infants, these drugs can cause abnormal movements, including seizure-like disorders, sluggishness, impaired respiration, growth retardation, and heart problems. Adding to the confusion and misdiagnosis, the neuroleptic drugs can also cause a worsening of the original gastric problems, including nausea and vomiting.

Tragically, some of these parents have been *convicted* of criminally abusing their children. Some have gone to jail and many have lost custody of their children as a result of being falsely accused of harming them. Ironically, the seemingly righteous doctors who accused them were unwittingly poisoning the children with neuroleptic or neuroleptic-like drugs.

The number of women falsely accused of poisoning their children may run into the hundreds. They have in common that their infants and children were treated with drugs like Reglan, Propulsid, Compazine, and Phenergan, commonly for gastric reflux. They are organizing and seeking legal representation. They can be located at a number of places on the Internet.

While the problem is not nearly as common in regard to children treated for ADHD, I have seen somewhat similar cases in which parents report the harmful effects of stimulant medication, such as abnormal movements or hallucinations, to the doctor and the doctor simply refuses to take the parents seriously or to believe them. The doctor then treats the parents as if they are irrational and irresponsible. In the extreme, the doctor or the school may call child-protection services when the parents refuse to continue the child on psychiatric drugs.

Tranquilizers and Other Sedatives

Especially after they have been overstimulated by Ritalin, Adderall, and similar drugs, children are frequently put on drugs to quiet them during the day or to induce sleep at night. Tranquilizers in the benzodiazepine class such as Klonopin, Valium, Serax, and Xanax are the most commonly prescribed. All of these drugs are highly addictive and can cause very serious withdrawal problems. They produce tolerance, requiring increased doses with increased risks. If stopped too abruptly, they can cause extreme anxiety, insomnia, and even seizures.

All of them can impair mental function. Combined with stimulants, all of them increase the risk of drug-induced out-of-control behavior. Xanax has a particular tendency to cause mania and violence.

A Potent Reminder of Drug Dangers

Versed (midazolam) is a very short-acting, extremely potent benzodiazepine that is used to relax and sedate children and adults for diagnostic procedures and prior to anesthesia for surgery. It not only reduces anxiety immediately ahead of time, it enhances anesthesia and causes amnesia for painful events. Unfortunately, Versed produces an extraordinarily high rate of abnormal mental and behavioral reactions during the several-hour recovery period and sometimes long afterward. In *Your Drug May Be Your Problem* (1999), I wrote, "Versed should be considered a very hazardous drug."

The dangers of the *pediatric dose form*, Versed syrup, recently caused the company to recall the product on an emergency basis. A precipitate in the bottle exposed the child to "a super- or subpotent dose" with the risk of "serious adverse health consequences or death." Roche Laboratories, the manufacturer, sent the notice entitled "Urgent: Voluntary Drug Recall" to physicians and health-care facilities by overnight delivery dated March 1, 2002. It arrived at my office on March 25, 2002, while I was finishing this book.

While not specific to the issues surrounding ADHD and stimulants, this recent event reminds us that FDA approval of a drug does not guarantee its safety. Caution is well advised concerning the use of any potent medication, especially those like Versed syrup with the potential to impair the central nervous system of children.

Mood Stabilizers

It has become a fad to diagnose children as bipolar, or manic-depressive, especially when psychiatric drugs have driven them into a disturbed or aggressive state. So-called mood stabilizers like lithium and Depakote, as well as a variety of anticonvulsant drugs, are used to smooth out the emotional ups and downs. In fact, they flatten emotional responsiveness and possess a variety of physical hazards. All of them cause ADHD-like symptoms, including cognitive deficits such as memory loss and difficulty focusing. Clonidine (Catapres) is too often given to children to sedate them. Combined with stimulants, it is a special hazard to the heart. If stopped abruptly, it can cause blood pressure to spike upward to a dangerous degree. The drug is used for the control of hypertension and is not FDA approved for psychiatric purposes.

This brief tour of psychiatric drugs is not intended to be an ultimate source of information. For more facts on the entire range of psychiatric drugs, you can read my book, *Your Drug May Be Your Problem: How and Why to Stop Taking Psychiatric Medications* (coauthored with David Cohen, 1999) or the *Physicians' Desk Reference,* which contains the FDA-approved labels. Keep in mind that all psychiatric drugs produce so many mental and physical abnormalities that no one source can cover them all.

The best policy in my professional judgment is to avoid giving psychiatric drugs to children. If children have already started taking them, the drugs should be used for the shortest possible duration. Stopping psychiatric drugs should be done carefully under supervision with an awareness of potential withdrawal problems.

Do "Alternative Treatments" Help with "ADHD"?

A huge industry has evolved around "alternative ADHD treatments." Vitamins and minerals, special foods and diets, complex dietary supplements, biofeedback, modified room lighting, tinted eyeglasses—the number of alternatives seems limited only by human imagination. These alternatives have in common that they address the physical functioning of the child's body rather than guiding the child's personal capacity to develop self-control and self-discipline. Some, like biofeedback, do encourage the child's capacity to take control, but they rely on gimmicks that are likely to make the child feel deficient and in need of special technological solutions.

Information about these alternatives is available from books, web sites, and magazine advertisements. Understandably, parents commonly turn to one or another of these alternatives in the hope of a less noxious alternative to stimulant drugs.

Reasons to Avoid Even "Harmless" Alternatives

Although most alternative interventions are not nearly as physically dangerous as stimulant drugs, they present some of the same psychological and moral hazards. They focus too much on the child and in particular on the child's bodily health. While children need to cooperate with their parents and teachers in learning to improve their attention and conduct, the focus should not be on them exclusively. All of the alternatives that I'm talking about focus on the child, and usually the child's body, as the source of the ADHD-like behaviors; but in reality, these alternatives do not address any proven or identifiable problem in the child.

The application of these various alternatives is likely to make the child feel "different" or even "abnormal." They undermine one of the most important lessons of life—that children and adults have the inherent capacity to learn self-discipline with the goal of accomplishing what they want in life.

These alternatives can distract parents and teachers from the key task of finding better ways to bring up and educate their children. Much like relying on stimulant drugs, turning to alternatives tends to disempower parents who should, instead, be developing their own parenting skills and finding new educational resources.

The Placebo Effect

Do alternatives sometimes work? Virtually every treatment in the field of human behavior at times seems to work. The most bizarre practices have their enthusiasts. Enthusiasm and hope—the placebo effect—will often have a temporarily good effect. The good effect results from the more optimistic expectations and perceptions of everyone involved, including the child, parent, teacher, or doctor.

The implementation of these alternatives usually requires increased parental attention and increased self-discipline on the part of the child. For example, getting your child to accept a diet free of food additives requires serious attention to your parenting and enormous cooperation from your child. As a result, many alternatives end up helping because they result in increased parental attention and cooperation from the youngster. However, the improvement comes at the cost of the parent and child understanding and consciously cultivating their real abilities.

Keeping Alternatives Available

Because most alternatives are not as dangerous as psychiatric drugs, I do not object to their use as strongly as I object to the prescription of stimulant drugs. In fact, I defend the right of people to sell and to use alternative treatments, and I agreed to work as a medical expert on behalf of a pharmaceutical company that sells an over-the-counter nutritional supplement.

The federal government was trying to stop the company from promoting its product as useful for ADHD. The substance has a mild stimulant effect similar to, but much less potent than, the classic stimulants. No serious adverse effects have turned up during controlled clinical trials or public use over a period of several decades. I effectively presented evidence that the supplement should be allowed on the market—even though I personally did not favor its use and would not recommend it to my own patients. In fact, I'm not even going to mention its name because I do not want to seem to endorse it. I bring it up to emphasize my belief that, unlike stimulant drugs, relatively harmless alternatives should remain readily available.

Genuine Physical Disorders

Real physical disorders can cause ADHD-like symptoms. If these medical problems impair brain function, they can make it harder for the child to impose self-discipline or to focus. But there's no evidence that children diagnosed with ADHD have subtle dietary deficiencies, biochemical imbalances in their brains, unique eye problems, or the like.

If children are suffering from eating disorders or languish in poverty and neglect, malnutrition can cause ADHD-like problems. Malnutrition of this magnitude is usually grossly obvious and does not require a hair analysis or other exotic diagnostic evaluation. Nor do these children need an expensive dietary supplement. They need three square meals a day and a multivitamin.

While there's no reason to suspect that many children with ADHD-like symptoms suffer from problems metabolizing sugar, common sense dictates that an overload of junk food is not healthy. Taking large bolts of sugar can result in a temporary rise and then a precipitous fall in the blood-sugar level, and the fall can produce transient hypoglycemia. Hypoglycemia can cause faintness, irritability, anxiety, and difficulty focusing. But these effects are temporary and rarely if ever play a role in causing persistent ADHD-like problems.[1]

Lead poisoning, head injuries, genuine disorders of hearing and sight, seizures, hypothyroidism, diabetes, sleep problems with chronic fatigue, chronic infections, heart disease, and brain tumors can interfere with the ability of a child or an adult to develop self-discipline or to focus. Many children take illicit drugs that cause them difficulties at home and in school. Others take psychiatric drugs that also interfere with their ability to control themselves or to focus.

From malnutrition to seizures, all of these children are suffering from known physical disorders rather than from "ADHD." While all children need regular medical evaluations, among the children treated for "ADHD," few are likely to have an undiagnosed underlying physical disorder as a significant source of their ADHD-like behaviors. Most of the exceptions involve children living in conditions of poverty and neglect.

Unfortunately, when children are suffering from real physical disorders such as lead poisoning, pediatricians, psychiatrists, and other medical doctors will too often fail to diagnose them in the rush to diagnose and treat "ADHD." As already emphasized, many medical doctors are especially prone to overlook problems that have been caused by their own prescription practices or those of their colleagues.

Educational Alternatives

Many supposedly ADHD children also have educational problems. As Chapter 14 discusses, these children do not have "learning disorders" any more than they have ADHD. But they do have gaps in their education—areas in which they have not been properly taught. Especially if a child cannot read well, school will be a difficult and unpleasant experience.

Tutors, peer teaching, and various remedial educational approaches can be helpful to children who need special help with the three R's. If they have widespread educational deficits, they may benefit from a new school or from home schooling.

Some computerized instructional programs seem useful for children who have missing links in their education, especially if they enjoy working alone and with computers. However, it can be difficult to find the right one for your particular child. From personal tutors to computerized math and reading curricula, parents need to take the time to learn about what's being offered by the program or the training course. Beware of any approach that promises too much, uses gimmicks, or claims to have identified a learning disability.

Chapters 13 and 14 address the nature of ADHD and learning disorders in more depth. For now, I want to reemphasize that in the absence of a real biological disorder, such as hypothyroidism or adverse drug effects, we should not blame the child's brain or body, and we should not direct treatment at the child's brain or body. Instead, we need to focus on improving the quality of the child's life, especially relationships with teachers, parents, and other adults. And when necessary we should provide special educational opportunities to fill gaps in schooling and to inspire an overall enthusiasm for learning.

The Ultimate Source
of Misinformation

Your doctor or pharmacist, the handout you were given at the drug store, the magazine article you read, even the books on drugs that you found at the bookstore and library—probably none of them offered the breadth of scientific information you have read in this book about the potentially harmful effects of stimulant drugs. You may have begun to wonder why the information contained in this book is not more readily available.

The subject of misinformation in the field of psychiatric medications is a large one.[1] I will focus on one key aspect of the problem—the lack of information contained in their FDA-approved official labels. These labels can be viewed as the ultimate source of much of the misinformation.

Where Doctors Get Their Data

Many and perhaps most doctors receive a large portion of their information about drugs from a combination of drug company representatives who visit their offices, drug-company ads and pamphlets, and the annual *Physicians' Desk Reference (PDR)*, which contains the official FDA-approved labels. Both the *PDR* and the sales reps arrive free of charge at the offices of nearly every physician in the country. The *PDR* comes once a year, but drug company reps come as often as the doctor can bear. And the drug company rep brings gifts of all kinds, from free drug samples for patients to free lunches, shows, and vacation trips for the doctors.

Practicing physicians are, of course, much too busy to review the overwhelmingly large literature on drugs that is churned out in professional journals. In addition to drug company salespersons and the *PDR*, they also rely on advertisements in magazines, reviews about drugs in various publications, and talks at meetings by other professionals.

From drug company reps to professional review articles, all of these sources are likely to be heavily influenced by the information in the FDA-approved drug label. When in doubt, the doctor will most probably turn directly to the handy *PDR* for the "official" scoop.

In part through my work as a medical expert in product liability cases against drug companies, I have learned a great deal about the creation of FDA-approved drug labels. These labels are at the heart of the drug-approval process. When the final label is approved, the drug is simultaneously approved for marketing.

For the basic scientific facts that go into the drug label, the FDA relies almost entirely on data generated by the drug company. The drug company meanwhile has complete control over the research. The drug company creates the rules for the research, selects and pays the researchers from among its stable of familiar preferred faces, and then collects all the data. Ultimately, drug company executives, rather than the researchers, prune and organize all of the study findings before sending them on to the FDA.

The FDA eventually reviews a small sample of the drug company data, asks questions, and tries to evaluate the overall safety and efficacy of the drug. Since the original data files are boxed in hundreds of large cartons and since the research has been conducted at multiple sites around the country, the FDA is hampered in conducting any kind of thorough monitoring. The agency has very little time or opportunity to check out the original data or the drug company's spin doctoring.

Nonetheless, the FDA usually finds many problems with the drug company's research and the data analysis, and begins to negotiate with the company about what to put in the label. In this negotiation, the government often lacks the resources or the will to overrule the interests of the drug company. In the end, the FDA-approved drug label usually turns out to be woefully inadequate and misleading in regard to both the effectiveness and the safety of psychiatric drugs. While the drug company and FDA remain responsible for updating these labels as more knowledge is accumulated, in reality the labels typically undergo very little change from year to year unless one or another potentially catastrophic adverse effect can no longer be ignored.

Remember tardive dyskinesia, that dreadful and yet common movement disorder that Alec endured as a result of treatment with the antipsychotic drug Risperdal? Tardive dyskinesia reports began to appear in the 1950s, but the FDA didn't insist upon a remotely satisfactory updating of the label until 1985. Even then, the FDA did so reluctantly under pressure generated by one of my books, *Psychiatric Drugs: Hazards to the Brain* (1983), and a Dan Rather TV report that the book inspired.

The Dexedrine and Adderall Labels

In regard to the all-important section on adverse psychiatric or mental effects, the FDA-approved amphetamine labels (Dexedrine, Adderall, and Adderall XR) are very weak and misleading.

Adderall and Adderall XR are products of a drug company named Shire US Inc. However, the adverse reactions part of the Adderall label is borrowed entirely and almost verbatim from the much earlier label for Dexedrine created by a different drug company, SmithKline Beecham. The 2002 Adderall and 2002 Dexedrine labels are *identical* for the critical section about psychiatric adverse effects:[2]

Psychotic episodes at recommended doses (rare), overstimulation, restlessness, dizziness, insomnia, euphoria, dyskinesia, dysphoria, tremor, headache, exacerbation of motor and phonic tics and Tourette's syndrome.

These skimpy descriptions, of course, in no way reflect the complete or even the necessary scientific knowledge concerning the many dangers of these drugs, including, for example, their enormous tendency to cause depression, sadness, tearfulness, apathy, and related depressed emotions in children. While it does mention several symptoms of overstimulation, it is also weak in regard to these drugs causing mania and manic-like symptoms such as excitation, agitation, and aggression. It entirely leaves out the production of obsessive-compulsive behaviors and overfocusing. There's no hint that the drugs can interfere with cognitive processes and learning. The observation that psychotic episodes are "rare" is simply false. "Rare" in FDA lingo means 1 in 10,000, when in reality psychotic reactions from stimulants are common (1 in 100 or more).

Indeed, the brand new 2001 Adderall XR label, which will probably appear for the first time in the 2003 *Physicians' Desk Reference*, drops the false claim that stimulant-induced psychotic episodes are rare. It refers to "Psychotic episodes at recommended doses." It's an improvement, but the Adderall XR label remains grossly insufficient in its failure to communicate the frequency of the risk.

The stimulant labels wholly neglect to point out that animal studies confirm that the drug works precisely by crushing spontaneity and causing apathy, submissiveness, and obsessive-compulsive disorder.

Finally, the labels say nothing about the numerous studies showing permanent brain damage in animals from exposure to clinical doses of amphetamine.

It is most extraordinary that the FDA allowed the Adderall label to borrow, word for word, from the Dexedrine label in regard to psychiatric adverse effects. Dexedrine was approved in the 1950s at a time when testing was very inadequate by modern standards. On top of that, there are differences between Dexedrine and Adderall that make Adderall potentially more dangerous. Dexedrine consists of only one chemical (d- or dextroamphetamine sulfate), whereas Adderall consists of four chemical variations of amphetamine.

How old is the portion of the Dexedrine label that was lifted verbatim into the Adderall label? Very. In regard to adverse psychiatric effects caused by stimulants, the Dexedrine label has been unchanged since 1984.

It gets worse. The 1984 updates were minor. In regard to psychiatric adverse effects, the 2001 labels for Dexedrine and Adderall actually go all the way back to the 1973 label for Dexedrine. The 1973 Dexedrine label read:

> Overstimulation, restlessness, dizziness, insomnia, euphoria, dysphoria, tremor, headache; rarely, psychotic episodes at recommended doses.

Thus, the only change between 1973 and 2001 was the addition of two neurological effects, "dyskinesia" and "exacerbation of motor and phonic tics and Tourette's syndrome." In regard to adverse psychiatric effects, there were no changes between 1973 and 2001 for the Dexedrine label and for the identical information copied into the Adderall label. That's twenty-eight years without a change, which failed to reflect the growing body of evidence during that time.

The Adderall XR Label

The label for the sustained release (longer-lasting) preparation of Adderall, called Adderall XR, came out in 2001 and will probably appear for the first time in the *Physicians' Desk Reference* in 2003.

The Adderall XR label has a section on amphetamine-induced psychiatric adverse reactions that contains a nearly identical copy of the old Dexedrine label going back to 1973. There's only one update. Psychotic episodes at recommended doses are no longer listed as rare. The word "rare" has been deleted. Remarkably, "rare" remains to this day in the labels for Dexedrine and Adderall. Physicians glancing at the Dexedrine and Adderall labels continue to be misled into believing that the drugs rarely cause psychotic episodes.

In addition to the twenty-eight-year-old observations on psychiatric adverse reactions, some new data have also been introduced into another part of the Adderall XR label. However, the source of the information is presented in such a confusing manner that a busy physician would rarely if ever have the time to disentangle it. Most important, a table has been added that shows adverse reactions derived from a "584 patient clinical study." The table is the first and perhaps only part of the label that will draw the busy reader's attention. The only psychiatric adverse reactions listed in the table are emotional lability [instability], insomnia, and nervousness.

Given what we know about stimulant drugs, one must immediately wonder about how the drug company managed to conduct a clinical trial for amphetamines that showed emotional lability, insomnia, and nervousness as the only psychiatric adverse reactions. It's not possible to tell from the table itself, but the answer is buried largely out of sight in the text of the Adderall XR label. The clinical trial used for the table lasted a mere three weeks.[3] Just three weeks! A three-week study is virtually useless for unearthing serious adverse effects in children who will be taking the drug for months and years.

A physician, researcher, writer, lecturer, parent, patient, or anyone else who turns to the "Adverse Reactions" sections of the current labels for the amphetamine stimulants is going to get drug company–spun information on adverse drug reactions that was already outdated in 1974. But in the case of Adderall XR, the reader might not get past the table, which is even worse in its failure to identify the dangers of these drugs.

The Ritalin Label

When I first wrote to the FDA to ask for the studies on which it based the approval of Ritalin in the 1950s, the FDA said they were lost. I was later able to locate them. Not surprisingly, these half-century-old studies were largely worthless, but they nonetheless continue to provide the basis for much of the official Ritalin label as found in the 2001 *Physicians' Desk Reference.*

At least the FDA required the Dexedrine label to utilize a new format implemented in the early 1970s. This revised format lists adverse drug effects under separate categories, such as "Central Nervous System" and "Skin," making it easier to read and understand. The Ritalin label for adverse drug effects still uses a single paragraph format that jumbles together all of the drug's harmful effects. Picking through the paragraph, we find only a few specifically psychiatric symptoms listed: "Nervousness and insomnia . . . anorexia . . . Toxic psychosis has been reported." "Transient depressed mood" is also listed, but with a disclaimer that no definite causal relationship has been established.

Compared to the Dexedrine and Adderall labels, the Ritalin label is even weaker. "Transient depressed mood" has been added, but overstimulation, restlessness, euphoria, and dysphoria have been left out, along with all of the adverse effects left out of the amphetamine labels.

How old are these data in the Ritalin label? In regard to psychiatric adverse effects, the 2001 Ritalin label reads word-for-word the way it did in 1973, except for the addition along the way of "transient depressed mood" with its associated disclaimer.

No wonder doctors, pharmacists, "informative pamphlets," and other sources are so weak in regard to describing adverse stimulant effects. Key portions of the official FDA-approved labels are based on decades-old material that was already skewed when it was put in the earlier labels for these drugs.

The Tip of the Label Iceberg

I have focused on the misleading and false presentation of facts about psychiatric adverse reactions in the FDA-approved stimulant labels; but this is a fraction of the overall inadequacies of these labels. The Ritalin label, for example, calls Ritalin a "mild" stimulant, when it is as strong and potentially dangerous as amphetamine and methamphetamine. The warning about addiction and abuse communicates that the problem lies in the addiction-prone patient and not the drug effect: "Ritalin should be given cautiously to emotionally unstable patients. . . ." The U.S. Drug Enforcement Administration (DEA 1995a, 1995b, 1995c), among other important sources, has repeatedly made clear that Ritalin is a very strong stimulant comparable to amphetamine, methamphetamine, and even cocaine (documented in Chapter 7).

The labels for stimulants are very misleading about the efficacy of the drugs. These drugs can do nothing more than suppress overall behavior, but they are presented as a specific treatment for a specific disorder, ADHD. Furthermore, while the lack of evidence for long-term safety and efficacy is mentioned, it is given insufficient importance. Physicians reading these caveats in the label would not be and are not discouraged from using the drugs long term.

What Allows for Such Disinformation?

There is a simple answer for why your physician and so many other sources don't have the kind of information contained in this book: Your physician and his or her major sources are relying on drug-company generated data that were already outdated and misleading more than twenty-five years ago.

Beyond this simple answer lie more complex forces, including open collaborations among powerful interest groups. There are hand-in-glove relationships among the drug companies, the FDA, and organized medicine. When I criticized drug-company support of the American Psychiatric Association in a letter published in the *New York Times*, the medical director of the association responded by stating that it has a "partnership" with the drug companies.[4] Recently, even establishment sources such as the *New England Journal of Medicine* have begun to publish criticism of drug-company control over research.[5] I have documented what I call the "Psychopharmaceutical Complex" in detail in books like *Toxic Psychiatry* (1991) and *Talking Back to Ritalin* (rev. ed., 2001a).

The public should pressure the FDA to take its mandate more seriously. The FDA should require drug companies to provide more accurate data on safety issues surrounding stimulant drugs. After all, we are giving these chemical agents to millions of our children.

Meanwhile, if our society treated its children with genuine care and concern, stimulant drugs would never have become FDA approved for the control of our children's behavior.

Chapter 13 focuses on the ADHD diagnosis that is used to justify the medicating of so many children.

PART II

Understanding and Improving ADHD-Like Behaviors

13

The Real Nature
of "ADHD"

Most people would be hesitant to give stimulant drugs like Ritalin and the amphetamines to children simply to make them more conforming or even to improve their academic performance. We have heard often enough about how wrong and dangerous it is for athletes to take stimulants, and it is also common knowledge that stimulants are abused on the street.

In order for doctors, parents, and teachers to accept the idea of giving stimulants to children, they have to be convinced that the drugs will treat a real or authentic medical problem. The more they can be convinced that ADHD has a proven biological or neurological basis, the more willing they will be to treat it medically. Promoting the concept of ADHD as a "neurobiological" disorder is key to promoting stimulant drugs.

The Limits of Current Neuroscience

At this point in neuroscience, how the brain functions is still beyond our comprehension. Despite advances in neuroscience, we still have very little understanding of how a single brain cell or neuron manages to respond to and transmit messages between itself and tens of thousands of other cells at the very same moment in time. On a biochemical and cellular level, we are at a very early stage of developing techniques for studying how the brain transmits messages. For example, we cannot measure the concentration of a single chemical messenger or neurotransmitter in the living human brain, let alone the overall functioning of the soup-like conglomeration of untold numbers of neurotransmitters acting all at once.

On a larger scale, we don't know what the organizational or operating principles are that result in what we call "mind" or "consciousness." We have little understanding of how the billions of cells and their trillions of connections actually create a functioning brain and mind.

Drug advocates have placed a great deal of emphasis on neurotransmitters; but many other forces also govern brain function. Some of the influences are gross, such as blood flow, oxygen consumption, and the availability of glucose. Other factors are subtle beyond our current understanding, such as the electrical forces that create patterns on the surface and deeper within the brain. Specialized cells of various kinds; numerous hormones; sodium, potassium, chloride, and innumerable other substances influence this complex organ.

Drug advocates frequently talk as if the functions of the brain and mind are dependent upon half a dozen neurotransmitters. In almost any textbook of psychiatry or psychopharmacology, they can be found speculating about the role of dopamine or serotonin in this or that psychiatric disorder. However, we know relatively little about how these neurotransmitters actually function. Furthermore, there are more than a hundred other neurotransmitters and related active substances in the brain, many of them as yet unidentified. And beyond that, we have no particular reason to believe that emotional reactions such as anxiety or depression, or problems such as inattention, are specifically caused by neurotransmitter dysfunction.

So why do experts indulge in these outlandish speculations about one or another neurotransmitter's role in psychiatric disorders such as ADHD? One reason is that the speculations make them look far more knowledgeable than they are. The speculations give them something to write about and a way to justify their grant requests. More important, drug companies routinely use these speculations to claim that their drugs correct biochemical imbalances. These absurd claims even find their way into television ads for antidepressants like Paxil.

Given our current state of knowledge, we have no real capacity to make scientific connections between brain function and the kind of complex mental phenomena and behavior such as the ADHD-like problems we deal with in everyday life and in psychiatry. The idea that "ADHD" is caused by a biochemical imbalance is sheer nonsense made up to justify the role of medically oriented experts and the use of drugs.

The Brain Scan Scam

In addition to their claims about biochemical imbalances, drug advocates also claim that children diagnosed with ADHD have "different brains" from other children. I have examined this fraudulent claim in Chapter 5 and in more detail in *Talking Back to Ritalin* (rev. ed., 2001a). Put simply, any abnormalities found in the brains of these children are far more likely to be the result of their exposure to psychiatric drugs. There is already a body of research documenting the harmful effects of stimulants, antidepressants,[1] and other psychiatric drugs on the brain. It is truly unconscionable to blame this medically caused brain damage on the child's "ADHD."

But There Must Be Something the Matter with These Children

Joey, age ten, seems like a kid who definitely has "something the matter with him." It seems like he cannot sit still. In a restaurant, he is always put on the outside of the booth so he can jump up whenever he needs to without climbing over everyone else. At the movies, he squirms around as if the seat is unbearably hot and ends up irritating people in a circle of seats around him. Several doctors have diagnosed Joey as displaying "classic ADHD," hyperactive type.

Joyce, age fifteen, daydreams in class. When asked to focus her attention on her work, she can only manage to do so for a scant few minutes at a time. She cannot remember to bring her books and homework assignments from school. At home, if asked to do a chore, she quickly loses track of her task and wanders off to do something else. She's been diagnosed as ADHD, the inattention type.

Harold, age nine, cannot seem to control himself. He's not only irritable, he will throw a temper tantrum the moment he is asked to behave himself or do a chore. In a group of children on a playground, he's always the one doing something "dumb" and getting into trouble. In class, he can't seem to control his desire to talk aloud any time he wants. At home, he's likely to grab something out of one of his parents' hands or knock over a fragile object on the table. He's been diagnosed as ADHD, the impulsive type.

George, age twelve, is a "completely out-of-control" child. He's the one described in ADHD books for parents as having an "engine running without brakes." In the last psychiatrist's office, he not only talked back every time he was asked a question, but he wouldn't sit still and ended up getting yelled at when he broke one of the doctor's vases. In school, he hardly ever pays attention to the teacher, but he notices everything else that goes on and causes a disturbance reacting to it. Even if another child starts the trouble, at this point George will be blamed for it. This fuels his constant complaints about being treated "unfairly." He's been diagnosed as ADHD with all three types. He's hyperactive, inattentive, and impulsive.

What Do These Children Have in Common?

What do Joey, Joyce, Harold, and George have in common? Biological psychiatrists and psychologists are likely to respond,

"They have ADHD in common. Each of these children has ADHD and each should be put on stimulants." They are also likely to declare that these children have a "biologically based disorder" or a "neurobiological disorder" caused by some as yet undetermined biochemical imbalance as well as by genetic factors. They would also show no surprise at hearing that all of them suffer from learning disorders, because those are often diagnosed along with ADHD.

Why ADHD Cannot Be a Biological Disorder

ADHD is not a "disease" that can be transmitted genetically and is in no way genetic; it's a description of behaviors that annoy adults and demand attention. As a recent review concluded, "ADHD genetic researchers cannot demonstrate that there is a convincing body of evidence pointing toward genetic factors."[2]

The very nature of the ADHD diagnosis renders absurd the hope of finding a common biological or genetic basis. The ADHD diagnosis is nothing more than a list of all the behaviors that annoy teachers and require extra attention in the classroom.

The list was developed over several decades by a core of drug-oriented professionals in order to justify the medicating of children who step out of line and don't conform to teacher expectations. If you doubt what I am saying, take a look at the criteria for the diagnosis as presented in the American Psychiatric Association's official *Diagnostic and Statistical Manual of Mental Disorders, IV-TR* (2000). They are reproduced in Table 13.1.

Key items in the diagnosis such as "often fidgets with hands or feet or squirms in seat," "often leaves seat in classroom," "often blurts out answers," and "often has difficulty waiting turn" have in common that they make life more difficult for teachers and other adults trying to manage groups of children.

Whether the behaviors are classified as hyperactive, impulsive, or inattentive, they have more causes than a single book could recount,[3] and nearly all of them lie outside the children themselves.

TABLE 13.1   Diagnostic Criteria for Attention-Deficit/ Hyperactivity Disorder

A. Either (1) or (2):

(1) six (or more) of the following symptoms of **inattention** have persisted for at least 6 months to a degree that is maladaptive and inconsistent with developmental level:

Inattention

(a) often fails to give close attention to details or makes careless mistakes in schoolwork, work or other activities

(b) often has difficulty sustaining attention in tasks or play activities

(c) often does not seem to listen when spoken to directly

(d) often does not follow through on instructions and fails to finish schoolwork, chores or duties in the workplace (not due to oppositional behavior or failure to understand instructions)

(e) often has difficulty organizing tasks and activities

(f) often avoids, dislikes, or is reluctant to engage in tasks that require sustained mental effort (such as schoolwork or homework)

(g) often loses things necessary for tasks or activities (e.g., toys, school assignments, pencils, books or tools)

(h) is often easily distracted by extraneous stimuli

(i) is often forgetful in daily activities

(2) six (or more) of the following symptoms of **hyperactivity-impulsivity** have persisted for at least 6 months to a degree that is maladaptive and inconsistent with developmental level:

Hyperactivity

(a) often fidgets with hands or feet or squirms in seat

(b) often leaves seat in classroom or in other situations in which remaining seated is expected

(c) often runs about or climbs excessively in situations in which it is inappropriate (in adolescents or adults, may be limited to subjective feelings of restlessness)

(d) often has difficulty playing or engaging in leisure activities quietly

(e) is often "on the go" or often acts as if "driven by a motor"

(f) often talks excessively

Impulsivity

(g) often blurts out answers before questions have been completed

(h) often has difficulty awaiting turn

(i) often interrupts or intrudes on others (e.g., butts into conversations or games)

B. Some hyperactive-impulsive or inattentive symptoms that caused impairment were present before age 7 years.

C. Some impairment from the symptoms is present in two or more settings (e.g., at school [or work] and at home).

D. There must be clear evidence of clinically significant impairment in social, academic or occupational functioning.

SOURCE: American Psychiatric Association, 2000. Reprinted with permission.

For example, these behaviors can result from any number of school problems, including unrealistic expectations for academic performance, unrealistic expectations for conformity in behavior, teacher frustration, student boredom, overly large and disorderly classrooms, and even abuse by other students.

Innumerable problems in the family such as anxiety generated by conflicts between the parents, lack of parental attention, and flawed or ambivalent parenting techniques can also lead to ADHD-like symptoms. Real physical disorders, such as lead poisoning, head injury, poor nutrition, exhaustion due to sleep problems, and an underactive thyroid can also contribute to a child's having difficulty with focus and attention.

Most commonly, these children simply have nothing wrong with them. They are displaying the normal behaviors of energetic children. ADHD is largely in the eye of the beholder. Too often, parents and teachers resort to blaming the child for requiring more attention and discipline than normal or for reacting to stresses in the adult world around them.

A list of behaviors with such diverse causes will never be found to be rooted in the mythical disorder called ADHD. Nor will behaviors like these ever be genuinely treatable with drugs. These children do not have something wrong in their brain, but rather in their lives.

In my own psychiatric practice, so-called ADHD children almost always turn out to be very capable of controlling their behaviors and disciplining themselves once their parents and teachers find the right approach to them and apply it consistently. That is, children labeled ADHD usually turn out to be entirely normal children living under out-of-control circumstances at home or in the school. They quickly improve as soon as the home and school begin to address their needs for discipline, love, and more-inspired education.

Some children labeled ADHD have never been properly disciplined in a consistent and rational manner. Some possess such rich and creative inner lives that they are bored and frustrated by confinement in a typical classroom. A few may suffer from genuine diseases, such as epilepsy or head injury, that cause them to seem inattentive at times. But none of them have "ADHD"—because that's not a disease or disorder, it's just a list of every kind of behavior that causes disruption or disorder in a classroom and requires extra adult attention.

Being diagnosed with ADHD doesn't automatically give these children anything in common, other than the very high likelihood of getting drugged.

Even the presence of very severe ADHD-like behaviors does not indicate a disorder in the child. The intensity of the behaviors instead depends upon the ability of the child's caregivers to meet the child's normal needs for such things as rational discipline, unconditional love, inspiring education, healthy peer experiences, exercise, and play.

In my clinical experience as a psychiatrist, many parents can be readily taught to relate to their children in more effective ways, leading to vast improvement in the child's behavior within a relatively short period of time. Sometimes, this can be done without the doctor working directly with the child. The changes in the parents bring about the changes in the child.

A Pernicious Diagnosis

Am I saying that ADHD is an essentially useless or meaningless diagnosis? Yes, that's what I'm saying. In regard to identifying or helping children, it is even worse than useless—it is very pernicious. It falsely blames the child for problems that have much more to do with the behavior of the adults in the child's life.

On the other hand, when a child is diagnosed as suffering from ADHD, it does tell us something about the professionals who are making the diagnosis. Most of them do not know how to provide genuine help to children, so they diagnose them as abnormal in order to justify medical interventions. Typically, these professionals suffer from a tragic inability to empathize with children, to understand the sources of their conflicts with adults, and to intervene in effective ways to help the adults overcome the conflicts. Moreover, by defining the symptoms of social stress and conflict as originating in a disorder in the child, the ADHD diagnosis directs the professional *not* to look for the real environmental causes. In my experience, doctors who specialize in diagnosing ADHD know especially little about the nature of adult-child conflict and how to resolve it in the home or classroom.

Am I saying that the diagnosis of ADHD tells us more about the experts than about the children they are diagnosing? Yes, exactly.

ADHD-Like Behaviors as Signals of Conflict

There is one thing that almost all "ADHD children" have in common: They are in conflict with one or more adults in their lives. The adults in the child's life have become sufficiently baffled, confused, or frustrated in their conflicts with the child to turn to experts for help. By the time they seek this help, they are often feeling completely overwhelmed by their child's behavior.

Unfortunately, when the experts make the ADHD diagnosis, it encourages the confused or frustrated parents to view these children as "beyond reach" by ordinary human means. In effect, the diagnosis labels the children as incorrigible and in need of extreme, nonhuman interventions, such as medication. It places the entire onus of the conflict on the child rather than on the more powerful adult. For the expert, it justifies drugging the weakest or most vulnerable member of the conflict. For the overwhelmed parent, it may provide temporary relief from feelings of guilt and inadequacy. Ultimately, this kind of resolution will do more harm than good.

When children are in severe conflict with adults, we must look to the adults as the solution. Children, on their own, don't have the capacity to resolve their conflicts with their parents and teachers. Conflict resolution between children and adults must be guided by the superior wisdom and maturity of the adults.

Helping the adults in the child's life to provide the child with proper guidance at home or in school can usually resolve the child's problems. This is especially true when the problems are at home rather than at school. Most parents are well-meaning; they simply need effective guidance from another adult, such as a counselor or from a parent-training workshop. When the problems are at school, some teachers may resist the idea that they have to change in order to meet the child's needs.

Because the ADHD diagnosis reflects conflict between adults and children, the diagnosis frequently depends on the tolerance level of the adults in the child's world. Some children "recover" from ADHD when switched from one teacher to another or from one school to another. Some recover when given over to the care of other relatives. Many do well on weekends and vacations or in classes or activities they enjoy.

Even when a child seems totally out of control, it doesn't change the nature or the solution of the problem. Even the most difficult and threatening child requires sustained, informed adult guidance.

Letting the Truth Slip Out in the Diagnostic Manual

In a surprising fashion, the official diagnostic manual of the American Psychiatric Association (1994, 2000) admits that ADHD is in large part a phenomenon that arises when adults aren't doing their jobs properly:

> Symptoms typically worsen in situations that require sustained attention or mental effort or that lack intrinsic appeal or novelty (e.g., listening to classroom teachers, doing class assignments, listening to or reading lengthy materials, or working on monotonous, repetitive tasks). Signs of the disorder may be *minimal or absent* when the person is under strict control, is in a novel setting, is engaged in especially interesting activities, is in a one-to-one situation (e.g., the clinician's office), or while the person experiences frequent rewards for appropriate behavior. (2000, pp. 86–87, italics added)

This paragraph contains a series of remarkable admissions.

1. The "symptoms" will appear or worsen in situations that "lack intrinsic appeal or novelty," i.e., that bore the child to death. But why should this be blamed on a disorder in the child rather than on the boredom of the classroom? Do we really want to label children mentally disordered because they don't respond in a docile fashion to "listening to classroom teachers, doing class assignments, listening to or reading lengthy materials, or working on monotonous, repetitive tasks"?

2. The symptoms will improve or even disappear and become "absent" when the child is in a "novel setting" or is "engaged in especially interesting activities." What can be concluded from this? A good classroom that engages and inspires children will eradicate ADHD from many a child's life.

3. The symptoms can also improve or disappear when the child is "in a one-to-one situation (e.g., the clinician's office)." How can this be? Many of these children are so starved for adult attention that their symptoms may disappear in response to the crumbs of attention they receive during a few minutes spent with a doctor. Most of these children are especially starved for one-to-one contact with a father or father-like person, so they are especially prone to behave well in the presence of a male doctor.

4. The "symptoms" will also improve or even disappear if the child is "under strict control." ADHD is a disease that can go away when the child is given sufficient discipline or supervision. Why is this? Because many of these children have never been given sufficiently strict control, or they have been given contradictory, inconsistent control that at times is overly restrictive.

5. The "symptoms" will also improve or even disappear when the child "experiences frequent rewards for appro-

priate behavior." What does this tell us? One of the most obvious principles of effective parenting—rewarding good behavior—is often sufficient to make this supposed disorder disappear.

This paragraph from the APA's *DSM-IV* contains, however unintentionally, much of the argument against the concept of ADHD. The "disorder" is not in the child but in the world around the child. As a result, the most obvious, effective, and honest way to remedy ADHD-like behaviors is to improve the world around the children, including our way of relating to them in the home and classroom.

These observations on ADHD in the diagnostic manual clearly indicate the situational or environmental nature of the "disorder," that is, its tendency to manifest in some situations or circumstances but not in others. Yet the label for Ritalin states, "Stimulants are not intended for use in the child who exhibits symptoms secondary to environmental factors." Thus, the description of ADHD in the diagnostic manual would rule out the use of drugs according to the FDA-approved label.[4] Contradictions like this are inevitable because ADHD is not really a disease or disorder and because drugs are not really an appropriate or effective response to the behaviors.

In Two Or More Settings

To shore up the case for ADHD, the APA diagnostic manual has added a caveat that the behavior has to appear in two or more settings. However, if a child is seemingly hyperactive, impulsive, or inattentive in more than one setting, it doesn't prove the child has a disorder. It could mean that the two settings have something in common. They may both be unruly, boring, or even threatening to the child.

Even if a child is behaving badly in many settings, or even all settings, it still doesn't justify diagnosing the child as the source of the problem. As I tell parents in my clinical practice, if your child is having a behavior problem everywhere, your child probably learned it at home. This is usually easy to show to the parents. Often the child was "difficult" even before starting school.

If the creators of the ADHD diagnosis had been more logical about it, they would have said that ADHD should not be diagnosed if the child is able to function more normally in *any* setting, such as a favorite class, on the athletic field, in front of the computer, or in the presence of particular adults.

Suppose a child has been diagnosed with a real disease, such as cerebral palsy (neurological impairments existing from birth) or muscular dystrophy (a degenerative disease of the muscles). We would be shocked to discover not only that the symptoms, such as abnormal movements or muscle weakness, disappeared but that the child became very physically able under certain conditions, such as when at home with parents, with a certain teacher or babysitter, on the ball field, or working with computers. In fact, if we did discover that the symptoms became "minimal or absent" under some circumstances, we would rejoice because it would probably mean our child didn't have a biological disease. We would, instead, look for psychological, social, or environmental causes that could be corrected.[5]

The disappearance of ADHD-like symptoms under some conditions is a strong signal that it is not a disease within the child's brain. Yet signs of hyperactivity, impulsivity, and inattention commonly disappear for periods of time and under special circumstances. In the more gross examples, sometimes they only appear in one teacher's classroom and at other times they will only appear with one parent.

In my clinical practice I sometimes find that a child is fine with one parent in my office but entirely out of control with the other parent. In my forensic work, I have testified in legal cases in which one of the parents tries to force the other to give drugs to a child, even though the other parent has no difficulty handling the youngster.

When the child's problems are rooted in the home, I explain to parents that it's very good news. If the problem began at home, it can be resolved at home with improved methods of relating to the child. I focus on helping the parents reach an agreement on basic principles of child rearing, and then I help them turn these principles into consistent practices.

The Hazards of Diagnosing Adult ADHD

When adults adopt the ADHD diagnosis for themselves, it can undermine their self-esteem and choice-making in a very self-defeating manner. Children are under the control of their parents and often trapped in boring, frustrating classrooms. But adults have more power to arrange their lives in a manner more consistent with their own true energy and interests.

Some adults with ADHD-like symptoms, such as poor concentration at work, may have had childhood experiences in their families or in school that have undermined their confidence in carrying out certain kinds of activities, especially those that remind them of "school." They may suffer from anxieties that were generated in the home or school. They may feel stupid and lack confidence. Or they may find it nearly impossible to do certain kinds of tasks, such as speaking in public or writing reports, because of earlier educational experiences.

These adults should not view themselves as having a handicap or disorder like ADHD requiring medication. Instead, they need to get at the root of their particular problems and find a useful, noninvasive solution that will not compromise the function of their brain with drugs.

Some adults with "ADHD" hate their jobs and wish they were doing something else, but they have no idea how to go about building their lives around what they love to do. They need to develop the confidence and obtain the guidance and information necessary to change their lives. Many can benefit from counseling or educational retraining.

Many other adults have a normal or even engaging personality that is restless and that resists confinement in an office. I often meet these interesting people in the media and in the legal profession. They frequently confess to me that by today's standards, they would have been drugged as children. They give a sigh of relief over having avoided that alternative.

In summary, the behaviors that we characterize as ADHD have an infinite variety of causes—from boring classrooms to poor discipline at home. Or they can be the normal response of an energetic child to situations that make unrealistic demands for conformity. Often children with ADHD-like behaviors have the capacity to become exceptionally creative and productive human beings. If they escape being diagnosed and drugged, and instead receive needed adult guidance, they can live unusually wonderful lives as children and adults.

The Real Nature of
"Learning Disorders"

Children are often diagnosed with learning disorders (LD). Many, if not most, children diagnosed with ADHD are also labeled LD. On occasion, I have seen children given stimulants in the hope of improving a "learning disorder." More often, the drugs are given for the combination of ADHD and LD, with the promise of improved academic performance. We are literally giving stimulants to children in the hope of improving their "performance." If this were openly done in regard to athletes, the doctor could lose his medical license and the athlete could lose the right to participate in sports.

What is a learning disorder? A learning disorder is identical to what parents and teachers in the past called "underachieving."

Before they have their child tested, parents almost always realize in advance that their child is "underachieving" in one or another academic area, such as reading, written expression, or math. That's why they seek professional help. When the parents are then told that the child has a "learning disorder," this information actually adds nothing to their original understanding of the problem. However, it raises the parents' anxiety level. It also raises false hopes that a problem has been properly identified and that the professional can offer a valuable service.

Underachieving: A Better Concept Than LD

Not long ago, a teacher could feel comfortable telling parents, "Johnny is underachieving. He's much brighter than his grades would indicate." Parents usually felt reassured to hear this. It meant he wasn't dumb—that he really could do better in school.

The LD Hoax

In the previous chapter, I described how the definition of ADHD is nothing more than a list of behaviors that disrupt classrooms. In effect, it's a kind of hoax.[1] LD is nothing more than an alternative way of defining and describing "underachievement." That makes it a hoax as well.

The latest edition of the *Diagnostic and Statistical Manual of Mental Disorders, IV* (2000) (*DSM-IV*) lists the official learning disorders as "Disorder of Written Expression," "Mathematics Disorder," "Reading Disorder," and the wastebasket "Not Otherwise Specified (NOS)." It points out that learning disorders were formerly called "Academic Skills Disorders." It then defines LD:

> Learning disorders are diagnosed when the individual's achievement on individually administered, standardized tests in reading, mathematics, or written expression is substantially below that expected for age, schooling, and level of intelligence.

In other words, your child will get diagnosed with LD if he or she is performing below expectation based on age, grade, or IQ.

If your child is ten but performs more like a typical eight-year-old on a standardized math test, your child has a math disorder. Or if your child is in the fourth grade and performs more like a second grader in math, your child has a math disorder. And finally, if your child performs above average on an IQ test but only gets average scores on a standardized math test, your child has a math disorder.

From the definition of learning disorder, you can see that I wasn't exaggerating when I said that LD is another word for underachievement. By definition, that's all it is.

Better to Be an Underachiever Than LD

Being labeled an "underachiever" had potentially positive, hopeful connotations. If nothing else, the child learned that he or she was not dumb or stupid. The "underachieving" child might be accused of being lazy or not caring, thereby earning a certain amount of disapproval. But the child wasn't accused of having a mental or physical defect, a permanent handicap in life.

By contrast, LD children by definition have something wrong with them. They can find themselves in the official manual of mental disorders. To make it worse, they are sometimes told that they have "crossed wires" or "biochemical imbalances" in their brains. Even if they are told, "You just have a different way of learning," it's not likely to add to their sense of potential or self-esteem.

An Outmoded, Flawed Concept

The LD diagnosis is usually made by comparing the child's performance on an IQ test to his or her performance on a standardized test of math, reading, or written expression. Also, variations within different functions of "intelligence," such as verbal or performance IQ, will be emphasized. This approach is based on the concept that there is such a thing as "general intelligence" and that specific deviations or variations from it are abnormal.

However, general intelligence, or IQ, has been highly controversial for decades. It assumes the existence of one generic intelligence factor and also focuses on rote kinds of activities learned in school. It has little or nothing to do with what I call *critical intelligence*, a concept that combines independence, wisdom, honesty, creativity, and courage.[2] As parents, critical intelligence is something we can cultivate by example in our children. If we do, they are likely to debunk ideas such as ADHD and LD.

Remember that IQ is not a physical entity in the brain that's visualized on a brain scan; it's a score on a pencil-and-paper test. Some children are good at test taking and some are not. Some children are so frightened about being "dumb" that they get flustered and perform poorly. Others think, "I can't do math," and their lackluster efforts prove them right. The tasks on the IQ test also favor children who are brought up in families that encourage and promote academic learning; therefore, enriching a child's environment can improve his or her "IQ."

Most important, the concept of general intelligence, or IQ, ignores the reality that "very bright" people are usually good at some things, such as reading and writing, but not so good at other things, such as math or mechanical puzzles. Vice versa, many people are good at math or mechanical puzzles and not at reading or written expression. As a result, modern scientists have discarded the concept of a general IQ and have replaced it with the concept of multiple intelligences.[3]

If we recognize that people naturally have a mixed basket of different abilities, then it makes no sense to label a child as disordered due to variations among the child's abilities. Like many concepts in biological psychiatry, LD is rooted in simpleminded, outmoded concepts that fail to recognize, among other things, human variation and the influences of environment.

Maintaining the LD Concept

What maintains this house of cards called LD? Money and professional identity. The concept of LD provides lucrative careers for many professionals. And like ADHD, it excuses the educational system from blame when it fails to teach the three R's. It is no coincidence that the concept of LD has grown at a time when our schools are being criticized for failing to teach reading, writing, and arithmetic.

The LD concept also preys on the fears and aspirations of parents who believe that their child must have every possible "advantage" in order to achieve in an increasingly competitive world. Professionals then mislead these parents into believing that success comes from being good at everything, when the fact is that success comes much more from being really good at one thing in particular and then having the courage to develop that ability with persistence and enthusiasm.

But He Reverses His Letters

Parents and other laypersons have been taught to believe that reversing letters when reading or writing is a sign of a learning disorder. In fact, years of research have failed to confirm letter reversal as anything other than a normal stage in learning. Some children stumble over this step, while other children never have a problem with it. If a child continues to reverse letters long after expected, the child needs additional help and practice—not a diagnosis.

Better Off Dumb?

If your child has a high IQ, it increases the likelihood of your child being diagnosed with an especially serious learning disorder. As a result, many bright youngsters are being saddled with the idea that they have something wrong with them.

How does this work? If your child performs far above average on tests of general IQ but for some reason only gets average scores on standardized math tests, then your child will be diagnosed with a math disorder. The existence and the degree of the disorder will be determined by the discrepancy between your child's general IQ score and the lower math score. Therefore, the "brighter" your child, the worse the disorder will be. By contrast, another child who gets average scores on both the IQ test and the math test will be viewed as normal rather than disordered.

As a result, many parents of very bright children are being told that their children have something the matter with them. This leads the parents to suffer enormous concern and anxiety, and to spend a great deal of time and money on remedial training. This, of course, can be very discouraging to both parents and children.

Many children would be better off if everyone thought of them as "average" rather than LD.

Problems with "Information Processing"

Wholly without scientific citations or other evidence, the *DSM-IV* (2000) suggests that some of the children labeled LD may have "underlying abnormalities in cognitive processing (e.g., deficits in visual perception, linguistic processes, attention, or memory, or a combination of these)." After opening this Pandora's box of psychobabble, the manual then adds a caveat: "Standardized tests to measure these processes are generally less reliable and valid than other psychoeducational tests." Unfortunately, the box has been opened, the caveat ignored.

Parents in droves are pushed to spend large sums of money to have their children tested for their supposedly specific learning problems. These parents become convinced that their children suffer from supposed impairments in "information processing," "sensory-motor integration," "auditory short-term memory," "categorical association reasoning," "inefficient planning and output," or "executive-regulatory functioning."

Many of these concepts were borrowed from earlier studies of grossly brain-damaged patients such as wounded soldiers, auto accident victims, and lobotomy patients. But these children do not have identifiable brain damage or dysfunction, and they have never been injured. These children are simply doing relatively poorly on one or another concocted test, with little or no proven relationship to real-life functioning.

The term "executive-regulatory functioning" has gained considerable currency lately. It is practically a fad. Parents are being taught by professional example to speak the phrase with reverence and, of course, to spend money to improve their child's executive-regulatory function. The term was originally developed to describe the central function of the frontal lobes of the brain. I find it ironically amusing that the language chosen to describe our highest human potential sounds like the job description of a corporate executive or government regulator.

When individuals suffer from severe injuries to the front of the brain from automobile accidents, gunshot wounds, lobotomy, electroshock treatment, or a lightning strike, they suffer impaired frontal lobe function. Under such tragic circumstances, they lose the kind of abilities that have been described as "executive-regulatory function," but they simultaneously lose an equivalent amount of their overall higher human functions, including the ability to use judgment, to be insightful, to make jokes, to enjoy beauty, to play, to empathize, and to love. In real life, so-called higher executive-regulatory functions cannot be separated from all of the other higher mental capacities.

When parents with children diagnosed with ADHD or LD are told that their children have problems with "executive-regulatory function" or some other cognitive ability, there is no evidence for real physical damage or dysfunction in the frontal lobes. Unless they have suffered a gross and obvious injury to the front of their brain, they don't suffer from a generalized loss of all of their higher human faculties. In fact, they have normal brains and normal brain function.

Making Things Even Worse

Children are sometimes put on psychiatric drugs in order to treat their "learning disorders." Based on the myth that stimulants improve educational achievement in children with ADHD, misinformed physicians imagine that drugs might help a child with one or another learning disorder. In reality, the stimulants impair mental processes and can produce a downward spiral in an otherwise normal child.

Recently I was consulted about a child who has permanent brain damage from psychiatric drugs. It all began with stimulants for a supposed learning disorder and then progressed to multiple psychiatric drugs.

Simon Says, "Move Your Right Arm"

When children are performing below their potential, it can be useful for teachers, parents, and the children themselves to recognize it. It's good news; it can be encouraging. The child has unused potential. Teachers may try harder to teach, parents may offer more encouragement, and the child may become more hopeful about doing better.

Mrs. Randolph taught third grade for twenty-three years, and for nineteen of those years, she volunteered each year to take on all of the readers in the third grade who were achieving below grade level. Why take on the most difficult kids? She explained, "Because that's where the teaching is. You can take the bright kids, hand them a book, and they'll do well. Teaching is helping the child who is reading on the second-grade level in the third grade."

According to Mrs. Randolph, "I would start out by talking with them and they had to answer me in a sentence. Not just 'Yeah' or 'Nah.' We would have conversations. These were the children who were not talked to at home. They didn't have language skills. So we talked. After all, how can you ask a child to read and to write a sentence if he can't speak it? So I taught them language. I taught spelling. I taught them about how to write a sentence. And this was all in the context of reading. I taught all kinds of skills: phonics [sounding words] as well as context [grasping a word through its context]. I taught them in any way that made sense to the particular child."

Many of the children could read words but lacked comprehension. She explained, "That's where my story reading would come in. They would sit on the floor around me as long as they didn't bother their neighbor while I was reading the story. That was always an underlying rule: You can't bother your neighbor. These kids are TV addicts. I would tell them to shut their eyes and imagine a TV. As I read the story, I'd ask them to imagine seeing the pictures in their mind's TV. Sometimes after reading, I'd have the children go back and draw what they saw. I would always read to these children interesting, easy books that they themselves could read or that were just a little above their level so that they could learn to read them."

Mrs. Randolph had some children with serious reversal problems. Many would write some of their letters backward, facing in the wrong direction. These children, she explained, typically did not know their right from their left. "I could help these children by playing Simon Says with them," she explained. "I would use instructions in the game that required learning to distinguish right from left." She adds with a knowing smile, "Knowing right from left also added to everyone's safety when they got old enough to drive."

Overall, Mrs. Randolph took a multiple approach to the needs of the child in order to reach the child and have the child comprehend. Sometimes she broke the children up into small working groups. "Often these were kids who were always alone in class and never had time to work together. I had them read aloud together in groups of twos and threes while I visited each group to see how the individuals were progressing."

In listening to Mrs. Randolph talk about teaching reading, it's clear that she thought a great deal about each individual child's learning problems and learning potential. I especially love the idea of her playing Simon Says with her children to help them burn off excess energy while learning their left from their right to overcome reversal problems.

In all of her years teaching children who were below grade level in reading, Mrs. Randolph never had a child whose reading didn't improve at least an extra grade level during the year. Many did even better, catching up to their peers. The children went, in her words, "from learning how to read to reading to learn."

Mrs. Randolph accomplished this without resorting to specialized psychological testing and diagnoses. She didn't frighten children and parents by talking about learning disorders characterized by faulty integrative functions or other pseudo-medical nonsense. Instead, she saw variation rather than pathology. She saw individuals in need of teaching rather than diagnostic categories. She identified each child's needs and used her imagination and skills to meet them.

Mrs. Holmes is a retired psychiatric nurse who doesn't believe in telling any children that they have something the matter with them that interferes with their ability to control themselves or to learn. She tells her Sunday school students they can do anything they want, as long as they are willing to put their minds to it. Then she guides and teaches them along the way to success. This fundamental idea—that with help from adults, children can do anything they are willing to put their minds to—is of course directly opposed to such concepts as ADHD and LD, which label children permanently handicapped.

We will meet Mrs. Randolph and Mrs. Holmes again when discussing more about how to provide guidance in the classroom (Chapter 18).

In conclusion, millions of parents are being bamboozled into thinking that they are getting a genuine service when they are told that their child has a learning disorder. In fact they are simply being told what they already knew—that their child is underachieving. Parents need to accept that children are inevitably good at some things but not at others. This, of course, is common sense, and it's been scientifically confirmed since the dawn of educational psychology. Now we've turned these natural differences into "disorders."

While it may at times be necessary to focus extra attention on a particular deficiency, such as reading below grade level, it remains essential to focus most of a child's time on the child's special abilities and interests. Otherwise, we create unhappy and frustrating lives for our children and discourage them from pursuing activities that will bring them satisfaction, joy, and success. Children and adults do not thrive on the basis of overcoming their deficiencies but on the basis of making the most of their strengths.

Allow your child to be gifted in one way but not another. Spend more time on encouraging your child's gifts and less time on focusing on his or her weaknesses. It will make for a happier and ultimately more successful youngster.

15

Why "ADHD" Should Not
Be Considered a Disability

ADHD has been designated a disability. Under Social Security, a child diagnosed with ADHD may merit a monthly check from the government that can be used in almost any way by the parent. Scandals have surrounded urban clinics that have encouraged impoverished parents to have their children diagnosed and medicated in order to obtain Social Security disability payments for ADHD.[1]

Under federal legislation and regulations, the ADHD diagnosis can lead to special accommodations in school or college, such as being allowed to take tests without being timed. It can also require schools to provide special services, such as smaller classes. Some states allow future professionals, such as aspiring lawyers, to take credentialing examinations without being timed if they have been diagnosed with ADHD.

Americans are generous and caring, and this has led our society to make many special accommodations for those who have disabilities. Blind people can now feel with the soles of their shoes when they are getting too close to the edge of a train platform because of the corrugated strip that lines it. A great deal of money was spent on this accommodation in order to make train stations safer for the blind.

Similarly, the sidewalks in my community have been modified at the corners to remove the cliff-like curbs. The curbs have been turned into smooth ramps to accommodate people with wheelchairs. The cement ramps also make it safer for people who have difficulty walking. It also makes it safer for children who come barreling along on their bikes and could easily get flipped over by a steep curb.

Accommodating disabilities can be a good thing. But should ADHD be considered a disability requiring accommodation?

In my practice, I have dealt with parents who wanted to maintain their children's ADHD diagnosis in order to enable them to take the SATs without being timed. Most colleges and universities require these grueling tests as a part of the application process. The SATs can easily become the most important examinations the high-school student will ever take. This, of course, makes the experience very stressful.

Preparatory courses for these tests always place a great deal of emphasis on making the best use of the limited time. Commonly, people don't finish these tests. Rarely do they have the time to check all their answers. If they could take these tests without any time limit, most people would do a great deal better.

Recently, I received a phone call from a judge who had previously asked me to give a seminar to his community on the overuse of psychiatric drugs for children. He was now concerned about accommodations being given for ADHD on the bar exam in his state. Applicants for a law license with an ADHD diagnosis were being allowed to take the test without being timed.

Why was this judge against allowing potential lawyers with "ADHD" to take as much time as they needed to finish the bar examination? He felt it allowed less competent attorneys to practice in his state.

It is ethically and sometimes legally wrong for professionals such as lawyers and physicians to practice while impaired. Indeed, it can be the duty of other professionals to prevent that person from practicing.

Presumably, the individual diagnosed with ADHD has sufficient difficulties with hyperactivity, impulsivity, and/or inattention to affect work. We know these individuals believe that it affects their test-taking ability. They may have trouble focusing on
details and tend to make careless mistakes in regard to details.
When in court, these individuals may have difficulty with emotional control. As someone who has appeared numerous times in
court, I know that some attorneys will do their best to get the op-
posing attorneys in the courtroom to "lose their cool" and to act
impulsively in front of the judge or jury.

It could be argued that speed in test taking has little relevance
to actual job performance in one or another profession. If state-
licensing agencies reach this conclusion, then they should not require any of the candidates to take timed tests. However, as long
as these agencies deem the tests to be of value as screening tools,
individuals should not be able to gain an advantage by claiming
to have ADHD as a disability. It is unfair to the other candidates
and not in the public interest.

The judge who brought these concerns to my attention said
that he had made an offer to compromise with the state board of
licensure. In effect, he said would go along with allowing individuals diagnosed with ADHD to take the bar exam without
being timed, providing that they received a special "ADHD license" to practice law. The license would have to be hung in a
prominent place in the office. It would say, "Warning: I have a
special ADHD accommodation. I may be slower, more poorly focused, and more impulsive than most attorneys, and you should
take this into consideration when hiring me or when agreeing to
an hourly fee schedule."

While the judge offered this somewhat in jest, he was also ex-
pressing his genuine concern about the danger of providing
ADHD accommodations in regard to activities, such as taking
the state boards, that might to some degree measure specific capacities that are advantageous or even necessary in the practice
of the law.

The issue of ADHD-like impairments was made very real to me when one of my friends, an attorney, received a head injury in a fall off a cliff while rock climbing. The injury left lasting impairments that are indistinguishable from so-called ADHD. Over a year or more, it became obvious to him that he could no longer focus with his accustomed intensity and ability. He had particular difficulty in organizing himself and in paying attention to details. Everything he did now took him extra time, but all of his extra effort did not result in a satisfactory result by his own standards.

Although none of his colleagues seemed to notice the change in him, he knew he was impaired and could no longer provide the quality of service that would meet his own standards for the practice of law. He decided to take a much less remunerative job, one in which the demands did not overwhelm his capacities.

The same issues can be raised about providing accommodations on the SAT tests used for college admission. Some of us are indeed much slower on tests. Should we be given an advantage in getting into college in a competition with other students who can work more rapidly?

Colleges now continue the ADHD accommodations, allowing these students to take tests, including final examinations, without being timed. This gives these students, self-identified as impaired, an advantage in getting good grades and hence in entering industries and professions that may require the very abilities that they lack.

While gaining an accommodation for test taking may give a youngster a competitive advantage over his or her peers, it can backfire by harming the individual's sense of personal worth. First, the individual is likely to realize that the advantage is unfair. Second, and perhaps more commonly, the youngster is likely to feel "impaired" by a mental disorder, biochemical imbalance, or genetic defect. Being "impaired" can be a dreadful blow to one's esteem when the impairment reflects a deficit in mental functioning. It would be far better for the youngster to feel "I'm terrible at test taking," or "I'm just slow on tests," or "I'm just not an academic whiz." Lots of people feel that way about themselves; but they have gone on to live highly creative and enjoyable lives that provide service and inspiration to others and that pay well. By contrast, a child who feels mentally impaired is not likely to have the self-confidence to live life as fully and successfully as possible.

I am not saying that people with ADHD-like problems cannot go on to become wonderful doctors or lawyers. Of course, many can; but some cannot. The only way to find out who can and who cannot succeed is to allow them to compete with everyone else on a level playing field.

The idea that ADHD is an impairment should be discarded along with the idea that ADHD is a disorder.

16

How to Provide Guidance in the Family

Psychiatric diagnoses and drugs, especially the stimulants, have replaced parenting and teaching skills. When we have a problem with the children in our care, we think of drugging them rather than guiding them.

It's time to revitalize the concept of guidance. Before we had "psychiatric" and "mental health clinics" for children, we had "child guidance" clinics. Noah Webster's 1856 *American Dictionary of the English Language* defines a guide as "one who directs another in his conduct or course of life" and illustrates the word "guidance" with this sentence: "Submit to the guidance of age and wisdom." Children need the leadership of age and wisdom. This simple truth has been lost amid the rush to diagnose and drug the children in our care.

There are many varied and effective approaches to helping children who display ADHD-like behaviors or other problems. All of them require adults to learn improved ways of raising and teaching children. Active opponents of the ADHD/stimulant approach have authored several good books.[1] There are also many other time-tested mainstays in the child-rearing literature.[2] No one has a monopoly on the best practices for raising children.

This chapter focuses on empowering parents to provide guidance to their children during the growing-up process.

Believing in Your Own Inherent Moral Authority

Nothing is more important to children than learning from the moral authority of their parents and teachers. Although the significance of moral authority seems to be missed by advocates of ADHD and stimulants, it is a central part of successfully raising and teaching children. Moral authority communicates the necessity of paying attention to important principles of living. Adults who have confidence in their own moral authority will be effective in creating respectful, productive relationships with children in the home, classroom, or playground.

Many of the children and families in my practice live in relatively affluent areas of Washington, D.C., and its suburbs. Although the nuclear family may or may not be intact, the parents are reasonably stable in their individual lives and usually have achieved a measure of success. However, by the time they come for help from an expert, most have given up trying to exert moral influence over their children and have begun to resort to a hodge-podge of threats and punishments, rewards and bribes. Often they are in such severe conflict with each other that they are undermining each other's authority with the children. My task is twofold: To reinspire each parent's sense of moral authority and to negotiate a common set of values in regard to raising the children.

Children Want Moral Guidance

When relationships have deteriorated, it seems like "listening to Mom and Dad" is the last thing a child wants to do. In reality, children cannot grow up in a normal fashion unless they respect the moral authority of the adults in their lives. As much as they sometimes resent it, children actually want their parents to possess moral authority.

Children do not feel secure making their own decisions on matters of great significance, especially in defiance of their parents. Instead, they usually feel terrified when they can "get away with it." They know that their ultimate safety and security comes from trusting their parents and having them in charge. Unfortunately, some families are in a state of such moral collapse or confusion that children are forced to find their own way. Sometimes they manage it remarkably well—but always at a great emotional cost.

Recovering Parental Authority

In the beginning of therapy, parents often need help in recovering their faith in their ability to influence the conduct of their children. They have lost hope of getting their children to listen, and their children, in turn, have given up listening. To the surprise of many parents, their children often welcome a renewed conviction that Mom and Dad expect to be heard with respect.

Radiating Rather Than Imposing Moral Authority

Your communication of moral authority is an extension of how you feel about and view yourself. Communication of moral authority begins with your personal conviction that you can and should create a respectful, loving environment in the home or classroom. You will radiate moral authority when you think of yourself as a rational, loving being who lives by principles worth communicating.

Children can walk into an unfamiliar home or classroom and know intuitively that they must behave respectfully in the presence of the new adults. Unfortunately, they can just as quickly sense that they are dealing with an adult who lacks moral authority.

In *The Heart of Being Helpful* (1997b), I describe the creation of healing presence—an inner comfort that allows your very presence to have a healing effect on others. When we create an environment of safety and trust around ourselves, others will find a corresponding comfort in our presence. In a similar way, when we become comfortable with our own moral authority and its rational and loving expression, we will radiate this authority when dealing with others in our lives, including children.

How Not to Influence Children

Yelling, screaming, threatening, and hitting do not increase a parent's or teacher's moral authority; they undermine it. The ability to implement humiliating punishments does not enhance moral authority.

When adults lose control over themselves, they also lose their influence over children. They may end up intimidating the children, but that won't help those children to grow up to be rational, caring people. When intimidated, children may outwardly conform, but at other times they will break into open rebellion or, even worse, withdraw into themselves.

Scaring a child actually undermines a child's ability to learn self-discipline by causing the child to obsessively focus on avoiding humiliation and injury. A frightened child becomes hyper-alert to the outside environment, and rational decision making is drowned out by the fears.

Too much reliance on rewards for good behavior can also undermine the child's sense of self-direction and the adult's moral authority. Children need to listen to their parents and teachers out of respect for them rather than in response to rewards and punishments. Punishment should usually be regarded as a signal of failure on the part of both the parents and the children. Parents need the confidence to take the lead in creating mutually respectful relationships without resorting to inducements or threats.

Children need to learn that good behavior or good grades is ultimately self-motivated and self-satisfying, and should be pursued regardless of rewards or punishments. In the real world of adulthood, our children will learn that bad behavior is often rewarded, while good behavior is sometimes punished. That's one of the reasons people have to struggle to live ethical lives; there are many forces encouraging us not to. To be prepared to live principled lives, children must learn to determine the direction of their conduct, based on good principles regardless of any immediate rewards or punishments.

Children Are Moral Beings

In my practice, when I talk with the children I'm treating, I relate to them as moral beings capable of reasoning with me about the kind of behavior that's genuinely in their own self-interest and about why one needs to learn self-control and empathy for others. As soon as children are verbal, and perhaps even before, they begin to develop a sense of right and wrong. At first, their moral sense is self-centered and their favorite complaint is "That's not fair." Soon, however, they begin to realize that something can be unfair to others as well. Similarly, at around the time that they become verbal, many children begin to show signs of empathy for others, including their playmates. They will toddle over to another child who looks sad to offer a toy, cookie, or hug.[3]

Sometimes I will talk to big brothers and sisters about how important they are to their little brothers and sisters. I will explain to a rambunctious boy that he is so strong that he can be gentle with other children. I will show a girl who fibs how telling lies makes it hard for her parents to take care of her. Sometimes I will use stories or anecdotes to illustrate a point.

I will also talk honestly with children about how their parents' conflicts or confusions have made it hard for them to know how to behave; but then I will emphasize that it remains up to them to become more responsible, regardless of their parents' behavior. I never assume that a child has a "disorder" such as ADHD or oppositional defiant disorder that renders the youngster unable to make ethical decisions and to exercise self-control.

Emphasizing Respect

When families show up for help, the adults and children have usually begun to lose respect for each other. Mutual ridicule and derision often mar the first few sessions. I point out the disrespectful nature of the verbal and nonverbal communications and explain that respectful communication is the single most important condition for improving relationships.

Once respectful communication has been restored or established, the family can begin to work on other issues, including conflicts about chores, homework, and bedtime. Until respectful communication takes place, none of those conflicts can be successfully resolved.

Sometimes more than their parents, children understand that everyone in the family needs to become more respectful toward each other. Sometimes the children let go of their negative behavior before the parents do. That's because the parents have been locked into their behaviors for decades, while the children have only recently learned theirs.

Mutual respect lies at the center of moral guidance. Parents too often try to demand respect from their children without first giving it. They lose control over their emotions, say humiliating or frightening things, and even hit their children in an impulsive manner. In their frustration, these parents have let outbursts of anger replace rational communication. That always creates a worsening situation.

When I counsel families with troubled and troubling children, I always emphasize the shared nature of the family problem. I emphasize the need for everyone, adults and children alike, to maintain respectful ways of relating to each other. To be respectful means to reach out toward the goodness in each other, to speak with kindness toward each other and, even when feeling emotionally injured, to avoid attempting to injure each other.

There are very practical implications to this emphasis on mutual respect. It means that speaking and acting respectfully toward each other becomes the central rule of the family. I urge parents not to conduct or to continue a conversation when the children are not being respectful. When communication becomes disrespectful, parents should stop the interaction, point out that nothing can be accomplished in an environment that lacks respect, and then begin again.

When respectful rules of relating are established, most other conflicts can be resolved in a mutually agreeable fashion. The children become more willing to listen to reasonable demands from their parents, and even to demands that may not seem so reasonable. They may even offer solutions of their own.

Love Is Not Enough—But It's Indispensable

Very loving parents have a head start in creating a happy, successful family life. Love is the stuff of life. Without it, a child withers and can even die. A loveless environment is poisonous to children.

I define love as a joyful awareness of another. Joyful awareness leads to treasuring and nurturing. I encourage parents and teachers to strive for an unconditional love that transcends momentary conflict and always pervades the relationship.

But love is insufficient by itself. I have worked with loving parents whose lack of moral authority encouraged their children to run rampant. The expression of love gradually becomes lost amid the chaos created by the now out-of-control children.

Respect sets the conditions in which love can most readily be shared. Therefore, I emphasize the creation of respectful relationships even before I focus on creating more loving relationships.

What About Discipline?

Blind obedience too often seems to be the goal of discipline. We want our children to be quiet and still on command, to study on command, to eat on command, and to go bed on command. Of course, we don't exactly put it that way, but in many ways it comes down to that.

Certainly, there are rare instances when small children should reflexively submit to the will of their parents. For example, a five-year-old needs to obey without hesitation when Mom shouts, "Don't run in the street!" or "Don't touch the hot stove!" But these are rare circumstances, usually involving matters of safety. Often they are the result of inattention to small children that places them in dangerous situations requiring emergency responses. A better approach is to keep a more watchful eye on small children in dangerous situations such as playing on the sidewalk or cooking in the kitchen.

In family life, respect is much to be preferred over blind obedience. If we teach our children to be respectful toward us and toward each other—that is, to relate in the family or the classroom with dignity, rationality, and caring—then we will have fewer problems with "discipline."

Seeking Professional Help

Parenting is the hardest job in the world, but parents receive little or no training for it. Good family counseling can be very helpful in honing one's skills as a parent.

In my own psychiatric practice, helping couples build happier families is among my most rewarding work. However, you need to screen professionals in advance on the phone to make sure that they don't favor diagnoses and drugs and instead offer a family approach.

Take your child to the pediatrician for the diagnosis and treatment of real physical disorders, such as hearing or hormonal problems that can interfere with self-control and learning; but don't rely on an ordinary pediatrician for opinions on child rearing or school problems. Nowadays, pediatricians usually have little time or motivation to do anything but diagnose and prescribe.

Insurance programs are willing to cover a ten- or fifteen-minute "med check" but not a full psychological and educational evaluation and ongoing counseling with the pediatrician. Physicians have adjusted their work to the exigencies of insurance coverage.

Seeking out the "best" in the medical field is not likely to be helpful either. If they have an appointment to a famous university such as Johns Hopkins or Harvard, they are very likely closely associated with drug companies and drug research. Some of the most biologically skewed work and fervent advocacy of drugs is done in these university medical settings.

The most effective professionals are likely to be counselors, clinical social workers, clinical psychologists, and family therapists. But even among them, too many have succumbed to the mythology of ADHD and drugs and to the search for "emerging" psychiatric problems. They are likely to end up referring your child to a physician for drugs. *You must check their views in advance, preferably by telephone.*

So Much for Preaching

Does it sound like I am preaching when I talk about moral guidance? Well, in a way, I am. Values lie at the heart of how we relate to our children. If we do not treat them with respect and love, we won't succeed in raising respectful, loving children.

Do I recommend preaching to our children? No, not generally. Preaching is more suited to addressing an audience in a book or in church. With children at home or in the classroom, we must above all else become personal examples of how to relate in a respectful and loving fashion.

17

How to Help
Out-of-Control Children

Most children diagnosed with ADHD and treated with stimulants do not have very severe emotional or behavioral problems. However, a small percentage of them are severely emotionally distressed, difficult to be around, and even potentially suicidal or violent. Usually their doctors have given them a second or third diagnosis such as the latest fad, bipolar (manic-depressive) disorder.

When I challenge the use of drugs to control children, the specter of the "really uncontrollable child" is often raised. References will sometimes be made to the existence of children who are like wild animals or monsters.

In my clinical experience, the more disturbed a child has become, the more the child needs, above all else, a consistent program of guidance in the home or, if necessary, in a protected setting. Stimulant drugs, like all psychiatric drugs, cause a disruption of the brain and mind that a distressed or disturbed child can ill afford. The child who is having trouble dealing with violent or self-destructive impulses or with hallucinatory experiences will be further confused by the unpredictable emotional impact of psychiatric drugs. Because stimulants, antidepressants, and other psychiatric drugs can cause adverse reactions such as depression and psychosis, it makes sense to avoid giving them to very disturbed children. As we have seen, the FDA-approved labels warn against giving stimulants to agitated and psychotic children. They also warn against giving them to depressed children. *Unfortunately, all potent psychoactive drugs, including all psychiatric drugs, can worsen the condition of a very disturbed child.*

Many of these children began with a diagnosis of ADHD and a prescription for stimulants. As I've already described, by the time their parents come to me for a consultation or treatment, the children are probably taking multiple psychiatric drugs, including especially dangerous antipsychotics like Mellaril, Haldol, Risperdal, Seroquel, Zyprexa, and Geodon. Commonly, the child's behavior has worsened a few weeks or months after starting each new drug.

These children are not "mentally ill," and they don't need drugs. They are simply out of control. Put more directly, their parents have lost control of their family life, and none of the half-dozen doctors who prescribed drugs have recognized the problem. This chapter is about regaining control of your family life and, in the process, teaching self-discipline and responsibility to your out-of-control child.

The goal is to create a rational, loving family life. While human nature doesn't allow for anything like perfection, parents can influence their family life in this direction and in the process help their children to mature without labeling them psychiatrically and injuring their brains with psychoactive drugs.

This chapter is an extension of the principles of guidance introduced in Chapter 16.

Parents at Odds with Each Other

By the time they arrive in my office for help with an out-of-control child, most parents are at each other's throats. Sometimes they are separated, and sometimes they are living together.

Typically, they began the marriage with somewhat different but equally valid approaches to child rearing. One parent started out with a healthy emphasis on nurturing but with a tendency toward being too lenient or permissive. By contrast, the other parent began with a healthy emphasis on consistent discipline but with a tendency to become too authoritarian. Either approach might have worked if applied with some consistency, but conflicts in the contrasting styles brought out the worst in each other and confused the child.

As the child became increasingly out of control, the parents became increasingly frustrated with each other and more polarized in their own attitudes, creating a vicious circle. Typically, the more permissive parent ends up blaming the child's misconduct on the other parent's authoritarianism and becomes still more permissive in an attempt to compensate. Conversely, the more authoritarian parent blames everything on the permissive parent, and becomes even more overbearing in an attempt to compensate. Both parents become increasingly angry at each other, often frightening each other and their children.

As the situation in the home deteriorates, a coalition is often built between the permissive parent and the out-of-control child, while the more authoritarian parent becomes isolated and increasingly frustrated.

At first glance, the more nurturing parent may seem "in the right," but in reality a vicious circle has resulted from the interaction between the two parents and the child's increasing tendency to manipulate the situation. As the parents grow angrier at each other, the marriage can be put at risk, while the child becomes increasingly upset and difficult.

To bring order to this chaos, the parents need to evolve a single consistent set of principles that aim at teaching responsibility and self-control to the child. Consistency in parenting, often more so than the specific mix of nurturing and discipline, is among the most critical aspects of regaining control of the family.

Of course, the scenario will vary a great deal from couple to couple, but these general principles are likely to hold: Parenting styles become exaggerated as the child's conduct worsens, leading to a vicious circle of deteriorating relationships and out-of-control behavior by the child. If allowed or encouraged, the child will manipulate the situation, often by siding with the more permissive parent.

A Parent at Odds with Herself

For simplicity's sake, this chapter focuses on families in which both parents are in the home. However, even when parents are separated or divorced, the same kinds of conflicts often develop between them around the children.

Furthermore, the principles remain basically the same when a single parent is raising the child. If only one parent is doing all the caretaking, the conflicts usually end up internalized within the one parent.

If you are a single parent, as conflicts grow worse with your child, one part of you will want to be permissive and may become overly lax at times. It seems temporarily easier. The other side of you will want to stop the bad behavior at any cost and will sometimes become outraged and even tyrannical.

As a result of your own internal conflicts, your child is confronted by the same kind of inconsistent parenting that can evolve in two-parent households. In response, your child may begin to manipulate you as if working two parents against each other. Your child will talk about your "good side" or appeal to your guilt feelings and try to get away with behavior that should never be permitted.

Your child will get your permissive side to agree to something that you really didn't want to do. When you later change your mind, your child will manipulate you as if you were two different people. "You promised" will replace "Dad said it was okay."

Eventually, your permissive side will become fed up with your more authoritarian side, your authoritarian side will become angry with your permissive side, you will swing to extremes, and for all intents and purposes, you're in a two-parent out-of-control situation. The solution, exactly as in the two-parent family, is to agree with yourself on a consistent set of rules and then implement them.

Trust Your Moral Authority

Read the earlier chapter on moral authority before reviewing the principles in this chapter. You must believe in your right to discipline and guide your child before you will be able to make any of these principles work.

Principles and Practices for Regaining Control of Family Life

The first several principles begin with the admonition "Do not. . . ." The key to putting order in your house is to stop behaviors that enable a child to remain out of control. When parents no longer reinforce negative behaviors, children will often spontaneously develop more satisfactory and mature approaches.

The following principles and practices must be adhered to without exception when a child is out of control. Otherwise, the youngster receives confusing communications and can manipulate the parents against each other. When a child becomes more consistently respectful, it's possible to be much more flexible.

What to Expect

When parents implement a more firm and consistent approach to dealing with a pre-teenager who is out of control, the child always begins to respond positively within a matter of days or weeks. While the same basic principles apply to dealing with the out-of-control teenager, they won't necessarily have the same immediate positive impact as on younger children, and additional interventions may be required (see below). School culture and peers become more important and add new stresses. Street drugs and alcohol can play a significantly harmful role.

Rules for Gaining Control over Your Family Life

On occasion, explain the following rules to your child. The change may at first seem confusing and even mysterious, and it helps to appeal to your child's rationality. Also briefly explain how the rules are in everyone's best interest but that they are especially intended to teach your child the self-discipline and personal responsibility that is required of all people. The explanations should be brief—limited to a few sentences. You should not discuss, debate, or argue about them.

Do not diagnose your child psychiatrically. Diagnosing and drugging children who are out of control almost always ends up worsening the situation. Diagnosing the child says in effect, "There's something the matter with you and not with us." The real problem is not the child but past parental failures to implement rational, respectful rules of conduct in the family. Trust that there's nothing the matter with your child that won't improve when you and your spouse work out your conflicts and agree upon a consistent plan for disciplining and raising your child.

In my own clinical practice, I usually spend much more time with the parents than the children. I don't find that diagnosing the children in the customary fashion is of much help, and I don't want to replace the parents as a caregiver. Instead, I try to help the parents "diagnose" the inconsistencies and conflicts in their parenting approach and in their marriage. As these conflicts are resolved, and as the parents learn to implement more rational and loving principles of child rearing, the lives of the children improve and the children begin maturing in a more normal fashion.

Do not become compliant or overreactive in response to the out-of-control child's disrespectful communications. Especially when parents are frustrated with each other, they may allow or subtly encourage the child's disrespectful communications toward the other parent. Establishing mutually respectful communication is the single most important principle in putting order into family life and eventually allowing love to flourish. When the child is screaming or yelling, the more nurturing parent is likely to make the mistake of saying, "Let him speak his mind," while the more authoritarian parent is likely to become danger-ously angry. Neither response is helpful.

The out-of-control child should learn to speak respectfully re-gardless of what he or she happens to feel at the moment. Re-member, that's the only way the child will be able to survive and then thrive in the outside world and in adulthood. Toward this end, the permissive parent must insist on respectful communicat-ing, even if the authoritarian parent seems to have gone over-board, and the stricter parent must exert self-control, even if feel-ing "over the edge."

Do not let the situation drive you into impulsive, angry acts. As the family situation becomes more chaotic, one or both parents are likely to become more impulsive. Typically, the more author-itarian parent may begin to ridicule and humiliate the child and the other parent. The more permissive parent may threaten to leave with the child. It is important for both parents to reestab-lish their own determination to relate respectfully toward each other and to demand the same of the child.

Do not "listen" to any communications that are disrespectful. When the child whines or speaks in an offensive tone or manner, both parents must insist on respectful communication before they respond in a positive way to the content of what the child is saying. If the child persists in speaking in an annoying or dis-respectful manner, terminate the conversation without giving in to any of the child's requests. Briefly explain your reason for ending the interchange but don't get caught up in "discussing" or arguing about it. In particular, never allow an out-of-control child to "get his or her way" by being difficult, obnoxious, or angry.

If the child becomes demanding, don't respond to the child's demands. Otherwise, you encourage demanding behavior. In-stead, tell the child to take time off in a place of his or her own choosing (not an enforced time-out) to cool down, and say that you'll listen when the child can speak respectfully and with concern for your feelings.

Do not accept the out-of-control child's tendency to blame someone else. When the child blames you or the other parent, respond this way, in effect: "It doesn't matter what we did; you were behaving provocatively and you are still behaving provocatively, and it's time to stop it." This brief explanation is sufficient and should not be discussed.

If you decide that you or your spouse also behaved inappropriately, discuss it with each other outside the child's hearing. While there might be exceptions, such as the need to intervene when the other parent is being abusive, avoid encouraging the out-of-control child's persistent attempts to blame someone else. At a later time, if you wish to acknowledge that Mom and Dad have made mistakes as well, do so without making it an excuse for the child's bad behavior. Remember, even if you're frustrated and angry with your husband or wife's behavior, your child needs to continue to learn personal responsibility under all circumstances.

Do not encourage out-of-control children to believe they have the same authority or influence as adults. Out-of-control children have often been allowed to feel unrealistically powerful or influential in the life of the family and may extend this attitude into the classroom and onto the playground. As a result, they do become powerful and influential, but in an entirely negative fashion.

While out-of-control children seem to want to be all-powerful, possessing too much power actually confuses and frightens children. Remind the out-of-control child that he or she is a child and is not in charge of the family.

In order to feel safe and secure, children need adult restraint and authority in their lives. Parents who emphasize nurturing at the expense of discipline can cause anxiety in their children. Conversely, parents who emphasize discipline at the cost of nurturing can also make a child feel unloved and abandoned and hence anxious.

Do not let the out-of-control child manipulate you against your spouse. Out-of-control children often try to get the "softer" or more permissive parent to take sides against the more disciplinary parent. The permissive parent will be tempted to blame the other parent for being too tough. Instead, focus on the out-of-control child's negative, provocative behavior. Tell your child, "It doesn't matter if Mom (or Dad) upset you, you still have to learn not to make things worse. If you won't control yourself right now, then take a break by yourself until you can behave with more respect and concern for us." Always emphasize to the provocative child that once he or she stops being provocative, the situation will calm down.

Remind the out-of-control child that the same behaviors that cause trouble in the home are also getting the child in trouble outside the home. Out-of-control children are so focused on the righteousness of their behavior that they have no idea it's unacceptable anywhere in life. It's a good idea periodically to remind your child that the behavior that must be stopped at home is the same behavior that must be stopped everywhere.

Emphasize the child's pattern of out-of-control behavior. Out-of-control children feel they are being treated very unfairly, and indeed they are; they have been deprived of consistent, rational parenting. However, they mistakenly think they're being treated unfairly when they are asked to get themselves under control.

Don't humiliate your children by reminding them of their past bad behaviors, but make clear that the current behaviors are part of an overall, long-term pattern that they must learn to stop. They may have been unfairly treated at times in the past, and even Mom and Dad may occasionally continue to treat them unfairly. But that's not the point. In the face of even unfair treatment, their behaviors make things worse for them and for everyone else. Furthermore, when they stop those behaviors, others will find it easier to treat them fairly.

It's easy to get trapped into particulars when dealing with the out-of-control child. Who started it? Who did what to whom? What really happened? If your child is behaving in a mature and rational fashion with you, these are, of course, important questions for discussion and explanation. But when a child has a serious pattern of disruptive, uncontrolled behavior, the pattern must remain the focus. Explain to your child that it will be much easier to deal with particulars when the overall pattern of behavior improves.

Don't get involved in arguments about what's fair with the out-of-control child.   It's worth repeating that the out-of-control child often feels unfairly treated. Indeed, parents, teachers, physicians, and peers often mistreat or unfairly blame out-of-control children. Explain to out-of-control children that their overall behavior—their pattern of behavior—tends to make people notice them and overreact to them, sometimes in an unfair manner. When the child gets under better control, there will be far fewer incidents of being treated unfairly. Make the explanation brief, and don't get tangled up discussing it.

Nothing in these principles should be taken to justify a parent becoming abusive or out of control.   A parent who teeters on the edge of losing emotional or physical control makes it much more difficult for the child to learn self-discipline and self-control. Beyond that, it's simply wrong to inflict our own emotional pain on our children, even if we think they've caused it.

Nothing in these principles should be taken to justify a parent's angry overreactions. Parenting does not provide us with an opportunity to vent or unleash; it gives us the opportunity to be as moral as we can in response to the sacred trust of raising our children. When you're feeling emotionally out of control, take a break, remind yourself that your job is to bring up your child in a rational and loving manner, and then return to implementing sound principles.

Helping Your Child to Stop Taking Illicit or Prescribed Drugs

Children who become involved with drugs and alcohol usually reject the influence of their parents and all other well-intentioned adults. The drugs interfere with the child's emotional ties and capacity to benefit from guidance. The peer drug culture usurps the family. In these situations, the parents need to intervene more actively to protect the child from harmful influences. It may be necessary, for example, to set more rigid restrictions on the child's behavior outside the home, to monitor the child's behavior outside the home, and to insist on drug testing as a part of the work of healing the family.

Prescribed psychiatric medications also interfere with a child's ability to connect to family and loved ones. They impair the child's emotional and physical maturation, and compromise the child's judgment, empathy, self-insight, and self-control.

The good news is that many children realize that the psychiatric drugs they are taking are doing more harm than good. Often, the child has reached this conclusion ahead of his or her parents and becomes the most enthusiastic supporter of drug withdrawal. The desire to give up the drugs can motivate the child to learn more responsible and self-disciplined behavior. The goal of being drug free encourages the child to both promise and make sincere efforts at self-improvement.

Chapter 8 deals further with the details and potential hazards of withdrawing from prescribed psychiatric drugs.

Be Alert for Abusive Relationships Outside the Family

Especially if parents are too busy outside the home or lack vigilance, even very young children can become involved in abusive relationships with other children or adults. Older children are prone to get involved in abusive romantic relationships, nasty cliques, or gangs. Much as you must do if your child becomes involved with street drugs, you may have to intervene to break up these relationships. Even if your child acts outraged over the intervention, he or she may be secretly grateful to have you interfere. However, in all cases it is best to rely at first on moral authority to influence the older youngster to let go of the abusive relationships.

Also keep in mind that teachers, ministers, youth group leaders, coaches, babysitters, and other authorities can be emotionally bullying or abusing your child. You may need to take actions such as intervening in the school situation or even changing schools or ball teams.

Assume Your Child Is a Moral Being

By the time they get to my office, at least one and sometimes both parents have ceased to believe that their child is a potentially rational and caring person. They no longer view their offspring as a moral being. As a result, they don't appeal to the child's natural sense of justice or to the child's empathy for others. Instead, they resort to anger and to punishments that are sufficiently extreme to worsen the situation and to further alienate the child. As the conflict worsens with the child, the parents feel more justified in deciding that the child lacks normal moral sentiments.

In reality, children often have a finer moral sensitivity than adults. Because they have not yet endured the many inevitable disappointments and disillusionments of adult life, they approach their own lives with a more naive and idealistic sense of right and wrong.

Throughout conflicts, always continue to appeal to your children's moral sense. Explain to them that their behavior is causing pain in others and that they themselves will feel happier when they bring more happiness to others. Explain to them how caring about the feelings of others will not only make them feel better but will achieve better results, and that it's also the right way to be.

Freely inform your child about the truth of how much better life becomes when we treat other human beings in a caring, ethical manner. And adhere to the standard yourself.

Taking Personal Responsibility for Ourselves

Taking personal responsibility for changing our own behavior as parents is the only way to break the vicious cycle of blaming each other. As a child becomes more out of control, parents typically escalate blaming each other. Each parent will overreact and exaggerate his or her own parenting styles in an attempt to compensate for what the other parent is doing. Thus, the more nurturing parent is likely to get excessively permissive and the more disciplinary parent is likely to get excessively rigid and overbearing. The parents then begin to undermine each other.

Of course, there are times when one parent must decide that another has become abusive and must be controlled or stopped. However, until the time that you decide to act to prevent abuse, try to see the problem as an interaction between you and your spouse that needs to be corrected for the benefit of all.

Unconditional Love

If you lose track of loving your child, the best principles and practices are still doomed to fail. The child will get the basic message, "I'm so bad even Mom and Dad don't love me." It's hard but important to do: Love your children as treasures in your care, even when you're stressed about imposing rational rules on them.

To prevent yourself from becoming impatient and angry with your child, keep in mind that your own parenting approach is partly responsible for your child's behavior. Also remind yourself

that it's your parental duty to teach self-discipline and responsibility and that ultimately you are giving your child a gift.

Your moral authority is based on your confidence in maintaining both a loving and firm attitude during your child's disruptive
behavior. Do not be afraid to feel love and to exercise discipline
at the same moment in time; this combination is the essence of
moral authority.

18

How to Provide Guidance in the Classroom and Other Groups

The principles of guidance that apply to home life also apply to dealing with groups of children, including students in a classroom. The teachers we will meet in this chapter have never advised putting one of their students on stimulants such as Ritalin or Adderall. They believe that drugs are not the way to try to help students with behavioral or academic problems in school.

At one time or another, many of us face the challenge of handling a group of rambunctious youngsters. Those of us who are parents get a taste of it at parties and outings that we organize for our children. One Friday night, when my youngest daughter was about fifteen, she had a party for about twenty-five of her friends at our home and everyone got snowed in together for three days. What could have become a nightmare turned out to be a wonderful time. Even the most rambunctious teenagers in the group managed to control their behavior out of respect for us as adults and out of appreciation for our providing an opportunity for a fun snow weekend. The boys had such a good time they volunteered to dig out our driveway at the end of the storm.

Even without being snowed in for a long weekend with two dozen teenagers, most of us at one time or another will be confronted with the potentially difficult if not trying task of being in charge of a group of children. Teachers, of course, are placed in this role almost every working day of their lives. Ministers, coaches, and scout leaders also end up having to deal with groups of children of various ages. The previous chapter looked at moral guidance in the home. This chapter focuses on the experiences of two classroom teachers.

Guidance cannot be offered to children the way a minister might preach a sermon to a congregation of adults. Guidance must be given more directly to children in response to their unique needs and differences. It requires paying a great deal of attention to each particular child. If that cannot be done, then there's something wrong with how the classroom or the group has been set up or is being run.

Guidance is not a matter of leading the group; it's a matter of taking individual children by the hand. It requires all of our capacity to empathize with the individual children and then all of our imagination to determine how to nurture each one's potential. Every teacher, parent, coach, or minister will approach the task with personal predispositions and abilities, so these examples can best serve as inspirations rather than as models to imitate.

Twenty-Three Years in the Third Grade

We met Mrs. Randolph briefly in Chapter 14 on learning disorders. Mrs. Randolph taught the third grade for twenty-three years. For most of those years, she volunteered to include in her classroom all of the "slow" readers from other third-grade classes. Class size in her Midwestern school varied from nineteen to thirty-one students. She taught until a few years ago and today remains active in education as president of her county's retired teachers' association.

Moral guidance starts with a moral purpose. For Mrs. Randolph, teaching was a calling. She spent many of her younger years volunteering in church and neighborhood activities and discovered her aptitude for working with children. As a stay-at-home mom while her children were young, she kept being drawn to the teaching field. It was as if a plan were unfolding that would lead ultimately to her teaching.

Although she taught well into the era of ADHD and stimulants, in most years none of her children were taking psychiatric medications. She never recommended that a child be given a medical evaluation or be given drugs and believes she never had a child in the classroom who needed drugs. Yet she was always assigned a disproportionate number of children that the school considered to have a "low aptitude" for learning. Listening to her descriptions of her children, it's also apparent that she usually had at least a few children who would ordinarily get diagnosed with ADHD or LD, or worse.

While her classes were sometimes larger than ideal, Mrs. Randolph always focused on individual children rather than on managing the group. She explained, "I took responsibility for every one of my children, no matter how many I had." She always tried to address the individual needs of every child in the class.

When Mrs. Randolph talks about her children, they come to life. She doesn't give the flavor of the classroom but rather the personalities of the individuals, many of whom she can recall in vivid detail years later. "Building rapport with each student is the most important task, especially finding out where each child is in his or her own learning curve. This cannot be done in a day. It's an ongoing process that is honed by the teacher."

In order to protect the children from being labeled or stigmatized, Mrs. Randolph never wrote down her evaluations of their needs, except in the most positive terms. Concerning their specific problems or seeming limitations, she kept only mental notes. "I didn't want my words to come back and be used against that child." This, of course, runs counter to the modern trend for many teachers and school psychologists, who seem eager to have children pigeonholed without regard for the harmful effects. "I wanted most of what I'd say to be positive so that someone else reading it could glean how to proceed in a constructive way with the child."

Every student was an individual. "I was not happy in the beginning of the school year unless on the first day I could call every child by name. And frequently as soon as I learned the child's first name, I would forget the child's last name. I didn't want to be influenced by family names that carried a history either positively or negatively. I wanted to deal with that young being in front of me to help him or her develop into the very best he or she could be."

Her approach to hyperactivity in children provides lessons that could benefit any teacher or parent. "With real behavior problems," Mrs. Randolph observed, "I've usually found they stemmed from the child having a need to move." Instead of seeking a drug to squelch this need to move, she tried to provide for its gratification. She would explain to the children that they would be allowed to have their own space in the corner of the room, "where they were allowed to do anything they needed to do to be comfortable with their body. If they had to get up to stretch that was fine. If they wanted to do an assignment in an unusual position, fine."

Mrs. Randolph described one little third-grade girl named Sue who liked to sit back on her spine, pull her knees to her chest, and prop her feet up on the desk. She wore dresses and that made her posture too revealing; but Mrs. Randolph didn't scold or ridicule her for it. Instead, she called Sue's mother and suggested that the little girl wear shorts or slacks under her dress so that she could sit in any position she wanted, and that solved the problem.

Mrs. Randolph explained, "Sue's mom was trying to make the child into a little lady and the child wasn't ready to be a little lady. Sue was very talented and her mind was going all the time. I made a contract with her that she would get her work done first and then she could get out her paper and write her poetry. If she wanted me to see her poetry, Sue could put it in a special place for me to find it. And for poems she didn't want to share with me, I gave her a private folder. I respected her wishes entirely."

Sue wasn't very neat and had trouble keeping track of a file folder, so Mrs. Randolph helped her stay organized. Meanwhile, Sue shared most of her poems with Mrs. Randolph, who was careful never to make a critical comment about them. "I kept her folder for her. At the end of the year, we took all of her poetry and bound it inside the cover she created to make a book which she took home."

Was Sue a special child getting special attention? Not really. Mrs. Randolph tried to discover and nurture the special qualities in each of her children. It was, from her viewpoint, her responsibility as a teacher.

Mrs. Randolph describes a boy, Mike, who was "very antsy, he was moving all the time, really hyper. So I put him at the back where he was given permission to move in any way he wanted, provided it didn't disturb the other children. He could get up, stretch, and move around in almost any way he wanted. He liked to work standing up, moving around the desk in a circle. By the time he got around the desk to his chair again, he'd be finished with the assignment."

Mrs. Randolph's description of Mike is offered with affection and even respect for his personal style of handling his energy. Nowadays, a teacher would be far more tempted to use this same description as justification for referring the child to a doctor for evaluation and medication.

Mrs. Randolph explained, "I treated Mike as a child with special physical needs and tried to meet his needs. He realized that he had that freedom to do what he wanted to do, as long as he wasn't disturbing someone else who was working."

I asked Mrs. Randolph, "What about people saying that Mike needed to learn to control himself—to stop himself from moving so much?"

Mrs. Randolph laughed and said, "Ah, forget it, he'll grow up and learn to control himself. He'll let it out in sports or elsewhere or grow out of it. Mostly it's boys with the excess energy. They'll find appropriate avenues in which to channel their own physical needs. And in so doing, they will discover their abilities, and be able to perfect those abilities, whether it's ball handling or teamwork. Many of these kids have leadership potential."

The approach taken by Mrs. Randolph requires a sometimes difficult balance between the needs of all the children and management of the group. But Mrs. Randolph never used the need for a quiet or orderly classroom as an excuse for taking suppressive measures against a child. At no point was she willing to sacrifice the child's needs for her convenience or for management purposes.

I asked Mrs. Randolph why so many teachers are willing to turn to diagnoses and drugs instead of innovative teaching approaches. She responded, "I don't think the young teachers of today are taught there is an alternative to drugs. And in all honesty, my system requires work. It takes effort. You're always thinking about a particular child. It's much easier to stand up in the front of the room with a predetermined idea of what you are going to do and then to teach the same lesson for the entire class." She is considering the possibility of teaching education students at her local university. "They really don't learn nowadays to relate to children as individuals," she explained.

Most of the time in the classroom, Mrs. Randolph worked one-on-one with individual children. "I would be up on my feet most of the day, walking up and down the class, checking how they were starting each assignment. I would take the child who was a little confused and walk him or her through the assignment. I was never happy unless every child started the assignment correctly."

This degree of individualized attention didn't leave Mrs. Randolph time to do all of the paperwork routinely required of teachers. "While the kids were in the classroom they had 100 percent of my attention." She often stayed after school to do the more bureaucratic work required of her as a teacher.

The children were allowed to converse with each other without permission, but they could not disturb or bother their neighbors.

If two children were both finished with their assignments, Mrs. Randolph maintained activity centers at the back of the room where they could go and talk, play a game, or do a puzzle. Sometimes they sat in twos or threes and just talked—children eight, nine, or ten years old enjoying each other's company. Mrs. Randolph explained, "Allowing children who finished to do more of what they wanted to do allowed me to work more one-on-one with children who needed my help."

Moral Authority Instead of Drugs

How did Mrs. Randolph accomplish so much with her children? I have been emphasizing her willingness and ability to accept children the way they are, even when they are hyperactive, and to create conditions in which they can grow to their fullest potential. But there's something else. Mrs. Randolph is a woman who commands respect. She possesses a natural dignity and can also bristle with a kind of no-nonsense sternness, especially when a child or adult offends her sense of common decency and mutual respect. She told me, "There was a lot of freedom in my class but it was *disciplined* freedom." I believe her; she radiates moral authority.

Mrs. Randolph always addressed her children with the moral authority of an adult who expects children to take her seriously. She believed in her own moral authority and conveyed it to her children.

Mrs. Randolph has very strong feelings against diagnosing and drugging children. As the medicating of children has escalated over the years, it's been apparent to her that the children put on drugs really needed increased attention from their parents and their teachers. Her years of experience as a teacher and as a mother of three have taught her that children need good parents and teachers, and that drugs are not the answer.

Twenty-Five Years in Drama and Still Going

Mr. Jackson has taught drama within a large and respected school system for twenty-five years at both the middle- and high-school levels. He has built one of the largest drama departments on the East Coast, and his shows often go on the road to other schools and communities.

It's an understatement to say that Mr. Jackson has a large following among the parents. He is adored by hundreds of them who feel that he rescued their children from educational oblivion, brought out the best in them, and helped guide them into productive lives. A surprising number have gone on to careers in acting or other areas of the theater, but others have transferred what they learned in drama to fields such as the law and teaching. As a young man, Mr. Jackson had a blossoming career as an actor but gave it up in favor of teaching.

When he walks down the street, you'd think Mr. Jackson was the mayor instead of the local drama and music teacher. Although he's not teaching in a small town, some people inevitably wave; others stop to say hello. There are stories to share about how his former pupils are doing. He not only remembers them, he knows their brothers and sisters, and sometimes even the family gossip. He's got a bearish and sometimes gruff manner; but it's easy to see through to the caring teacher.

Mr. Jackson told me that his own experiences in elementary and high school were very painful, he was not a good student, and he was only "saved" by the confidence and interest shown in him by his drama teacher. He believes that his personal background has made him willing to reach out to more difficult students.

On the surface, Mr. Jackson and Mrs. Randolph are very different people. Mrs. Randolph looks like a pillar of the family and community who'd be at home at a bake sale for the church. Mr. Jackson looks like a former athlete who'd rather be hiking in the mountains or hunting in the fields.

But they have a great deal in common. Both love the children they have taught and continue to know or to teach. Both are aware of the family lives of many of their students. Both take great pride in their teaching and have worked very hard at it for many years. Both see students as individuals and are much more concerned about the potential of each one than about maintaining order in the classroom.

Both found it natural to focus on individuals while maintaining order in a group. Mrs. Randolph may do it with a chiding glance and Mr. Jackson with an occasional bellow, but they each share an absolute conviction that they should be in charge of their classrooms and that that they should do so by using a combination of caring and unflagging discipline. Both see themselves as adults helping children rather than as the children's buddies or friends.

Most striking to me, however, is the vividness with which each of them brings their children to life in the stories they tell about them. They really care about the individuals. This, to me, is the core of the art of teaching. I've been a classroom teacher at several universities, but I have spent only a fraction of my time teaching compared to my full-time practice of psychiatry. Mrs. Randolph and Mr. Jackson are able to care about individual students in a way I could never manage in a classroom or other group setting. I have to be in the safer and more intimate surroundings of my own office in order to focus with such interest on the individual. They manage to accomplish this in the classroom and, in Mr. Jackson's instance, even amid the chaos of a large theater production. That makes them great teachers.

Increasing Teacher Stresses

Like Mrs. Randolph, Mr. Jackson is totally against the use of psychiatric diagnoses and drugs. He simply doesn't think of a child as "ADHD" or "LD" and would never want to see a child taking psychiatric drugs. He has refused to fill out the ADHD forms that get sent around to evaluate individual children, and on a couple of occasions, he's taken the risk of letting parents know that their child had been unable to participate fully as a result of the dulling effects of medication. He tells me that he can often watch the children nod off or stare into space, and he knows then that they've just been to the nursing office for their afternoon dose.

Mr. Jackson doesn't think that children diagnosed with ADHD are stigmatized nowadays. Instead, he finds that they use their "disorder" as an excuse. They will tell him, "I can't learn that script, I'm ADHD" or "I can't stop tapping my foot, I've got ADHD." Youngsters also tell him, "I can't do that today because I forgot to take my medication." The diagnosis and the drugs, he fears, are undermining the personal responsibility of teenagers and fostering excuse making that will impair their growth and development.

Does Mr. Jackson have it easy as a drama teacher? Does he get highly motivated students who are relatively free of problems? While he does get many highly motivated students, he also gets more than his share of the "problem kids." Some end up in drama when they have been forced to drop out of a regular class and need something to fill in the slot. Some are drawn to him as a potential father figure. Parents have been known to push their troubled children to take drama with Mr. Jackson.

I asked Mr. Jackson why there's so much more reliance today in the schools on diagnosing and drugging children. He doesn't think it's driven by the teachers themselves but rather by the conditions under which they have had to teach in recent years.

In the affluent suburbs, Mr. Jackson observes, many students will never be able to achieve on the level of their highly successful parents. The parents want "the best" for their children and even want them to succeed a step beyond themselves. But often this will be unattainable for many of the young people in their communities. As a result, parents and then teachers place unrealistic pressures on them. This leads to pressure to diagnose and medicate the children to improve their performance.

Today's teachers, he further explains, have far greater stresses on them. For example, they are expected to be available on demand to parents and administrators alike. Parents often want to be able to reach them by e-mail, pager, and cell phone. While there's some advantage to ready contact between parents and teachers, it can also be very trying for the teachers.

Mr. Jackson observes that the schools have become much more overcrowded in the last ten years. While class size has not substantially increased in his school district, there's a need to fill every single space in the school with activities all of the time, with the result that there's less time or place for leisure. Teachers also have to teach a greater number of classes and end up working longer hours. The schools are larger, making them less warm and caring places. The teacher shortage and the use of untrained, inexperienced teachers adds to the stress level for everyone.

Grading is more frequent nowadays, and paperwork has also increased massively. Everything has to be documented. It leaves less time to devote to teaching or to enjoy it.

Then there are the new standards of learning tests that are used to monitor the progress of students and their teachers. If the students don't perform up to par on the tests, the heat is put on the teachers. While this doesn't have a direct impact on Mr. Jackson as a drama teacher, it does increase the overall tension in the school.

But probably the biggest problem, in Mr. Jackson's experience, is the lack of respect for authority on the part of students. Mr. Jackson attributes some of the disrespect for authority to the breakdown of family life and family values. Parents find themselves unable to control their own children or to teach them respect.

Some of the problem flows from a general downgrading of the authority of teachers in society. Years ago, parents would almost invariably side with the teacher, whereas nowadays they are more likely to side with their children. Even school administrators have lost their authority and live in fear of lawsuits when they consider disciplining a child.

In part due to the breakdown of adult authority, violence in the schools is increasing, and many have hired security guards to patrol the halls and handle fights. Racial tensions are sometimes high. Cliques add to the atmosphere of hostility.

As someone who found public school too confining, Mr. Jackson feels that today's young people have an even more difficult time because there's even less time given to activities that provide an outlet for their physical energy or imaginations. When they arrive in his drama class, he explains, "They come to me as if they've just been let of prison. All day long they've had no outlets where they can have freedom to move around outside the classroom." He'd like to see more time allotted to physical activities, as well as to programs and projects that involve more active learning and community activities.

Throughout the years, Mr. Jackson has managed to maintain his own moral authority in the classroom, but it comes at the cost of increasing stress. Ten years ago, he loved teaching much more than he does today. Some of the change he attributes to his own aging process, but I don't believe that's the problem. Under better circumstances, he would now be a patriarch enjoying great respect in the classroom and school.

In sum, teaching has simply become too stressful. Even the best teachers are feeling the strain. Diagnosing and drugging the children as if they are to blame makes no more sense than diagnosing and drugging the teachers into submissive conformity with the declining conditions in our schools. Neither the teachers nor the students are to blame, and the students should not be psychiatrically turned into scapegoats for the failings of the school system, family, and society.

Traveling America

When I travel, I take the opportunity to see what people are thinking who seem to have nothing to do with the issues that preoccupy my life. To my frequent surprise, I find that most people are touched in one way or another by psychiatric diagnoses and drugs, and it often involves children. To my gratification, they usually don't like the increasing drugging of America's children.

On one of my trips, I sat for nearly nine hours on a train next to Mrs. Holmes, a registered nurse from Georgia who spent much of her career working in a mental hospital that treated children and adults. She now teaches Sunday school. I introduced her briefly in the chapter on learning disorders. She is the woman who believes that children should not be told that they have a disorder that interferes with their ability to control themselves or learn.

In the opinion of this experienced psychiatric nurse and teacher, if a child cannot concentrate or behave, it's not a psychiatric problem. Such children shouldn't have their self-esteem injured by being sent to psychiatrists. Instead, she finds that parents and teachers can reach any child if they try hard enough and in the right way. Her own approach is a mixture of common sense, good parenting and teaching, and religious inspiration.

I asked Mrs. Holmes why her approach works when so many other teachers are convinced that numerous children need medical intervention. She answered, "I think it's a matter of patience—understanding and listening to the child. Often the child can tell you more than you can learn by just watching them. And most of the time you can take what they say and turn the negative into a positive." She gives the example of children who complain, "I hate math." She tries to build up their confidence. "I explain to them, 'Maybe you hate it because you're not understanding it.' And then I help them with their math. If they say the teacher is teaching too fast, I tell them to ask the teacher for a little extra time and I'll help them too. All they need is confidence in themselves that they can do it."

"All children are different," she believes, "And some won't ever concentrate on school the way other children do." She also finds that many children who don't seem to be listening are in fact taking everything in. Mrs. Holmes had a granddaughter who used to stand on her head in pre-K, and the teacher would tell Mrs. Holmes that her granddaughter had a problem. But then one day the teacher asked the youngster to explain what she'd learned while standing on her head, and it turned out she'd been absorbing everything.

While Mrs. Holmes believes that adults must exert authority in their relationships with children, she never scares or intimidates the children. She told me, "Any child can be reached and making them fearful doesn't do any good."

As long as a health professional or a teacher harbors the idea that some children cannot be reached, then some children will not be reached. It becomes too easy to justify diagnosing and drugging the child who challenges us instead of searching deeper within ourselves for the personal resources required to reach a particularly difficult child. The concept that "any child can be reached" is key to the approach taken by successful mental-health professionals and teachers as well as parents.

Mrs. Holmes is not shy about telling people that children don't need stimulant drugs. She had a little boy in her Sunday school class who was taking Ritalin, and she discouraged his parents from continuing with it. She believes the ten-year-old was out of control in the classroom because he could not read and because he did not believe in his ability to read. "I told him he can learn to read—that he just had to put his mind to it. I helped him to learn to read and to pronounce the words. He needed confidence and now he's doing much better without ever needing drugs."

The people I meet who understand that children don't need diagnoses and drugs always recognize that children do need dedicated adults in their lives to provide them with moral and spiritual guidance. As parents, these people feel that children are a sacred trust. As professionals, they feel they have a calling to work with children. They feel comfortable and enjoy providing psychological, moral, spiritual, and educational guidance to children.

As I described in *Reclaiming Our Children* (2000a), we must make the kinds of changes that are needed, including better-trained teachers, more interesting curricula, more time and space for physical activity, and school policies based on respect for teacher and student alike. In the meantime, parents and teachers, much like Mrs. Randolph and Mr. Jackson, will continue to do their best to meet the needs of their individual children. But the public needs to rally to the cause of making our schools better places for our teachers and our children.

19

When the School Says Your Child Has a Problem

This book emphasizes the importance of your moral authority as a parent or teacher dealing with children at home and in the classroom. Now comes the great test of your parental authority—how to react when the school declares that your child has ADHD or LD and needs a medical evaluation that will probably lead to stimulant drugs.

When we are told that our child has a "problem" in school, terror often strikes our hearts. Short of a medical specialist's diagnosing a life-threatening physical illness, few things are as distressing as being told that our child has a "mental" or an "educational" disorder.

Nowadays, parental fears are often reinforced by dire warnings that if untreated, our child is likely to have a clouded future. If we respond by seeking a medical or psychological consultation, our worst fears may be amplified by unfounded predictions such as: "Children with ADHD have a higher rate of school failure, delinquency, and drug addiction." While we reel under these bleak predictions, our doctor is then likely to describe stimulant medication as if it were a harmless panacea capable of warding off all of these potential tragedies.

Given the fears engendered by teachers and health professionals and the corresponding offer of a panacea in the form of medication, no wonder millions of Americans overcome their intu-
itive distrust of psychiatric drugs and end up going along with a
prescription for Adderall, Ritalin, or some other stimulant. And
when parents do resist drugging their children, it's no wonder
that teachers and professionals, and even the courts, will sometimes seek to force them to comply.

While recent state legislation has begun to discourage and even to
prohibit teachers and other school representatives from specifically
recommending medication, school authorities can still recommend
a "medical evaluation," with its inevitable prescription of drugs.

What are parents to do when the school brings up a "problem"
that seems destined to lead to psychiatric medication? Most important, remind yourself of your moral authority as a parent. Be
prepared to continue to guide your child's life not only at home but
also in dealing with the school. Beyond that, your approach will
vary from circumstance to circumstance, but for discussion purposes we can divide up the problem into several overlapping steps.

Step 1: Find out what the teacher or the school is thinking.
Although there may or may not be any truth to the teacher's or
the school's conclusions, be open to hearing their observations.
Ask the teachers to describe their concerns in detail so that you
can make an independent evaluation. If it turns out there's little
or nothing to it, you'll be more able to respond effectively.

In my own clinical experience, most children singled out by
teachers for "medical evaluation" simply need more attention
than the school is willing or able to provide them. The child is
blamed for the school's inability to respond to the child's needs.
On the other hand, some children do have serious problems that
may interfere with teaching them in almost any setting.

Step 2: Make your own evaluation of the school's observations.
You will want to talk with your child about what's going on at

school. You may want to visit the classroom to observe for yourself. If your child is said to have a "learning disorder," you need to decide for yourself whether your child really has educational gaps that require special help. In most cases, your child's academic record and your own observations should suffice to determine whether your child is simply a little slower than other kids in one phase or another in learning, or very bored, or too curious and imaginative for the classroom, or in need of a tutor to fill in some gaps. Seeking help from an educational consultant should be done with grave caution; too many of them are part and parcel of the ADHD/Ritalin establishment.

Step 3: Make a serious evaluation of your child's conduct and attitudes outside the classroom. Evaluate how your child is doing at home, at church or scouts, during sports or other recreational activities, at the computer, with babysitters and relatives, and in public in stores or restaurants. Ask for impressions from friends who have spent time with your child. Try to determine whether your child seems as happy as most other children and, if not, what circumstances he or she finds especially distressing. Your next steps will depend on whether or not you think your child is having problems outside of school.

Step 4: What to do when your child has difficulties at school but not at home. If your child is doing well at home and in most other situations, you can focus your attention on the "school problem." Many different factors can make an otherwise self-disciplined and happy child seem maladjusted at school.

Many of the nation's classrooms are too boring for a child with any real imagination and energy. Your child may not have a particularly tolerant, able, or inspiring teacher, but even so, it might be possible to encourage the teacher to meet more of your child's needs. The school may have resources, for example, a guidance counselor who can work with you, your child, and the teacher. In the extreme, it may be possible to change teachers or schools.

Even if your child behaves wonderfully outside of school, you should visit the classroom. You may discover that your youngster is out of control in class. Even if you cannot figure out the reasons for this, you may be able to help your child learn to settle down and pay better attention.

Although the problem is showing up in the classroom, it may originate elsewhere at school or even on the way to school on the street or in the bus. Children often suffer extreme peer abuse. Many get teased and ridiculed on a daily basis. Some are physically and sexually threatened most of the days of their lives at school. Your child may have difficulty telling you anything about this, but if your child seems frightened about going to school, become alert for peer abuse.[1]

You may need to consider a variety of alternatives, from a change of schools to home schooling.[2] Children diagnosed with ADHD in the eyes of one teacher can turn out to be delightfully welcome in another's. Some children who seem to hate school can prosper in a school that meets their needs or in well-organized home schooling.

Many children don't like school and never will. If that's the case, you should still try to find or create the best possible environment for your child, including home schooling. In addition, you need to do everything you can to encourage and enhance any and all of your child's interests, from photography to computers to dance and sports. Some of these activities may be available in school or through your county. Try to spend interesting and enlightening times with your child by going together to the movies, museums, or theater, and by camping, hiking, or traveling together. As your child reaches the teenage years, seek out informal or formal internships for your child in interesting business and professional activities.

Step 5: What to do if your child is also having problems outside of school. If your child has behavior problems at home as well as at school, it's time for self-reflection as a parent and for seeking ways to improve your parenting skills. If a child is a constant stress to be around or seems very unhappy, then there is something wrong in that child's life, and home is the first place to look.

Some common problems include fathers who aren't involved enough in a child's life, parents who are in personal conflict with each other in the home or who have separated, parents who cannot agree upon how to raise the child, an abusive parent, and parents who are too rigid or too lenient.

Sometimes experiences outside the home can be so traumatic that the child will be disturbed in many areas of life, including at home. In very young children in particular, be aware of the potential for sexual and emotional abuse at the hands of anyone with power over your child, including teachers, coaches, ministers and other clergy, babysitters, and peers at school.

In Chapters 16 and 17, I have provided an introduction to some of the basic approaches to regaining control over your family life and helping your child develop self-discipline and personal responsibility. Also remember that any good bookstore has shelves filled with books keyed to helping parents with bringing up their children.

If you decide to seek counseling, keep in mind the warnings and suggestions I have offered in Chapter 16 about making sure to pick someone who shares your values.

Step 6: Taking a stand with the school.   While always seeking a cooperative and friendly relationship with teachers and other school authorities, it is important to maintain your moral authority and decision-making rights. Remind yourself that you are the parent and that you have a moral right (if not a legal right) to resist any and all efforts to diagnose and drug your child. However, in most situations there's no need to come on strong at the beginning. That's why I've left this section for last. Only in the extreme should you let the school know that you're digging in your heels concerning the diagnosing and drugging of your child and that you won't tolerate it.

As pleasantly as possible, remind the school that you will not pursue medication solutions and that you do not want your child given "psychological" or "behavioral" tests. Tell them you're sure that the usual academic achievement tests given to all children will suffice for your child as well. At the same time, make clear your intention to work with the school in every other way. To reassure the school, you can explain that you will seek any needed psychological evaluations on a private basis.

Especially if you are being pushed against your wishes toward having your child evaluated or medicated, you may want to seek legal help. There are lawyers who specialize in helping parents get what they need from schools. I have been called on to testify as a medical expert in a number of cases that have resulted in schools backing off. However, the best policy is always to begin with an open mind toward what the school is saying, coupled with your personal determination to remain in charge of your own family life and to make your own health decisions for your child.

Getting Worse
Before It Gets Better

There are positive signs of a "Ritalin backlash." A number of states are taking countermeasures by passing legislation that prohibits teachers from talking to parents about psychiatric diagnoses or medications, or the presumed need for them.[1] The controversy continues to heat up as the media casts an increasingly skeptical eye on the massive drugging of America's children. Increasing numbers of books are coming out that raise doubts about using stimulants and offer alternatives. Where once I seemed like a relatively lone voice, many professionals are now speaking out against diagnosing and medicating children.

Unfortunately, despite these positive signs, the drugging continues to escalate. Stimulant sales probably surpassed $1 billion per year in 2001 as the drug companies became more aggressive. In August 2001, Metadate, a long-acting form of methylphenidate (Ritalin), was advertised in the back-to-school issue of such magazines as the *Ladies' Home Journal*. McNeil Consumer Health Care, which makes Concerta (another long-acting methylphenidate preparation), and Shire US Inc., which makes Adderall (an amphetamine mixture), have also been advertising directly to the public, but without mentioning the name of their product. McNeil has run sixty-second TV ads on such networks as the Discovery Channel and A&E.

In the past, at the urging of the U.S. Drug Enforcement Administration, the pharmaceutical companies have respected international treaties that prohibit advertising these highly addictive stimulants directly to the public.[2]

Among the nation's 50 million school-age children, 4–6 million are probably being exposed at any given time to stimulant drugs, and the number is growing.[3] In addition, an undetermined number of adults are also taking these medications for the same purpose of treating ADHD.

Studies have shown that that at least 15–20 percent of fourth- and fifth-grade *boys* in public schools are receiving these drugs,[4] and the figures have almost surely risen in the last year or two. Even larger percentages of children are taking psychiatric drugs in individual public and private schools. Surveys indicate that *most* children in foster care and other social service programs are being administered psychiatric drugs. In special classes and in schools that specialize in learning or behavioral problems, most or even *all* of the children will receive psychiatric diagnoses and drugs.

Furthermore, increasing numbers of preschoolers, including children one or two years old, are being diagnosed and medicated. In all cases, these very young children are receiving drugs that have not been approved for their age group. Often, they are receiving drugs that have only been approved for adults.

Even if we assume a conservative figure such as 4 million children taking stimulants at any one time, the number by no means reflects the scope of the problem. Consider these additional implications:

- To the several million children who are taking stimulants at this moment, we need to add the millions of others who have taken these drugs in the past and the millions more who will take them in the near future. With the continued introduction of new stimulant drugs backed by increasingly aggressive advertising, the numbers of children will continue to grow. For the indefinite future, a very substantial and growing portion of our children will be raised on stimulant drugs for months and years at a time.

- Because prescribed stimulant use is so widespread, children and adults get the idea that the drugs are relatively harmless, and therefore begin to obtain and to use them on their own. The widespread prescription of the drugs also makes them more freely available for this kind of illegal use.

- Stimulants do not correct "biochemical imbalances"— they cause them. As a result, many children who have been treated with prescribed stimulants will turn to illegal stimulants such as cocaine when they reach their later teens or early adulthood. It's a simple fact that stimulants alter the normal functioning of the brain. Therefore, many youngsters will find a continuing need for them.

- In addition to the physical risks inherent in taking psychoactive drugs, these children are being influenced by the idea that they have mental disorders. They are taught that they have "attention deficit hyperactivity disorder" as a result of "crossed wires" or a "biochemical imbalance" in their brains. For the remainder of their lives, they are likely to see themselves as partially disabled or handicapped, if not "defective" or "mentally ill." They will feel psychologically incapable of overcoming these supposed "disabilities." Instead of learning greater self-control and self-discipline, they may become lifetime consumers of psychiatric medication.

- Beyond the effect on the individual children who become labeled and treated, there is a larger impact on schoolchildren in general, all of whom are now growing up in an environment in which children who fail to meet adult expectations are being diagnosed and drugged. In effect, all of our children are being exposed to a new set of family and school values that define "difficult" or even "disappointing" children as fit for psychiatric diagnosis and drug treatment.

• The diagnoses and drugs not only change the children, they change the caregivers. When a child nowadays shows signs of conflict with adults in any setting from the school to the church, concerned adults are encouraged to believe that they lack the personal or professional skills to help the child and that drugs must be introduced into the child's life. Parents, teachers, and health professionals have lost faith in their personal ability to provide adequate parenting, teaching, and counseling to the children in their care. The widespread use of psychiatric diagnoses and drugs has undermined the confidence and ability of everyone who tries to take responsibility for contributing to the lives of children in the professional office, home, classroom, or community.

• The children who are being diagnosed often represent our most energetic, individualistic, and creative youngsters. They are the ones who require the extra attention that our schools and families often feel unable to provide. Our diagnoses and drugs are in effect pruning a generation of our children by medically subduing any who stand out in ways that test our patience and skills. As a result, we are permanently impairing and undermining many of the children who would otherwise grow up to take leadership positions in our society.

• Because we have defined so many children as suffering from "learning disorders" and "ADHD," we have lost the motivation to reform our schools and to improve our families and communities on behalf of all children. We have become a child-blaming society. While this lets us off the hook of responsibility for our children, it robs us of our most sacred responsibility—to continue to evaluate and to improve the conditions under which our children grow up. It deprives us of the satisfaction of knowing that we have taken full responsibility for the care of children.

• Many children have "graduated" from stimulants to combinations of other psychiatric drugs called "antidepressants," "tranquilizers," "mood stabilizers," and "antipsychotic drugs." Often, these drugs are given in an attempt to control the adverse effects of the stimulants. By the time I get to see these children in my psychiatric practice, the parents have forgotten that their children were originally given stimulants for relatively benign problems, such as daydreaming in class or failing to do homework. Their more serious behavioral and educational problems actually evolved during the stimulant treatment and then worsened with the addition of each new drug. Now that their children are taking two, three, four, or even five psychiatric drugs at once, these parents are dismayed to realize that their children were in fact doing much better before any of the drugs were started.

• There are many additional costs associated with diagnosing and drugging children, including hundreds of millions of dollars spent by families on medications and on consultations and treatment with ADHD advocates. School systems, communities, and state and federal agencies spend multimillions more of the taxpayers' money for special programs that encourage drug treatment.[5] Often these treatments create additional problems for the child, including stigmatization and adverse drug effects that require hospitalization. These add to the cost of medical and psychological treatment. Although drug advocates often make unproven claims that their treatment will reduce the overall financial cost of helping children, the staggering cost of "diagnosing" and "treating" so-called ADHD is almost never counted or addressed.

- Finally, the widespread use of psychiatric diagnoses and drugs has weakened the foundations of society. While this statement might at first seem extreme, it is not. The foundations of any society are based upon how it views and treats its children. Western culture has been built upon the idea that the vast majority of children, perhaps even all children, have the capacity to respond to proper discipline, unconditional love, and education. We now believe instead that millions of children, including most of the children in special classes and schools, are essentially incorrigible—unreachable by ordinary human intervention. These children, we now believe, must be given psychiatric labels and subjected to psychoactive agents. It may take generations for us to begin to grasp in retrospect the extent of the damage this approach has inflicted on the basic values and principles of our society. Tragically, much of the damage will go unrecognized in the form of lives that never fulfill their potential.

The final chapter finds hope in the future for America's children.

After September 11—
A Better Future for
Our Children

Since the tragic terrorist attacks on our nation, our views of almost every aspect of life have taken on a different coloration. Many have voiced the feeling that nothing will ever be quite the same again. Certainly, the positive aspects of growing up and living in America will not be so easily taken for granted.

Perhaps these events will wake us up to the necessity of promoting strength and courage in our children. We may begin to realize the self-defeating nature of subduing our brightest, bravest, and most energetic children with Ritalin, Concerta, Adderall, and the growing armamentarium of psychiatric drugs.

Until September 11, we didn't think much about the kind of courage and perseverance our children might need to survive and prosper as young men and women in the future. Perhaps because life seemed so relatively easy for us as adults in America, we hoped to make it equally as easy for our children by whittling away their rough edges and smoothing them into acceptable shapes. We used to hope that a "well-rounded" child would roll along into a future free of deep crevices or high hills. Those hopes no longer seem so realistic.

In easier times, we anticipated that unemployment would remain low and that job opportunities would remain high as our children grew up. For the time being at least, that expectation has been turned on its head. All of a sudden there's job insecurity in our own adult lives, and we can no longer feel quite so secure about the future careers of our children. Our children might need to learn a degree of toughness and determination to handle future uncertainties.

We used to imagine that our economic prosperity would continue for the foreseeable future. Our children would continue to benefit not only from our own investments but also from theirs. Now many of us feel anxious about hanging onto the money we've already earned.

We used to imagine that living in the United States was relatively safe, especially in comparison to the rest of the world. In regard to our children, we were more concerned about the fears engendered in them from watching movies than from watching news coverage of events in our own nation. Now we feel the need, on the one hand, to shield our children from real life and, on the other, to prepare them for actual warfare.

We used to want our children to grow up to learn science and medicine mostly for their own satisfaction and success and perhaps to contribute to humankind as well. We had licked smallpox—we could lick almost anything. Now our society may need these scientific and medical skills for its very survival, even against smallpox.

We used to think that getting along was more important than integrity, and we were willing to encourage our children to adjust to existing conditions. In a world filled with uncertainties and in need of leadership, we may make more room for the expression of our children's critical intelligence.

We used to shun making value judgments about other cultures. While still favoring pluralistic values, we can also see the necessity of taking a strong stand against the victimization of women, children, and entire societies when perpetrated in the name of religious or national fervor. Like our forefathers, we are once again recognizing the existence of universal human rights. We may find ourselves talking more with our children about principles and how to live by them.

We used to think it was enough to be sensitive and aware, and to get along with other people. Now we accept our government's call for us to be alert and brave, ready to fight. We see the need for honoring heroic police officers, firefighters, and soldiers. We are witnessing the revival of a concept of "manhood" that had fallen into disrepute during times of relative safety and ease.

It's not clear yet how these changes will affect the way we view, raise, and educate our children. But we can hope, as in other areas, that the recent challenges will mobilize us in new and better ways as a community.

We can hope to see that it's a dead end to force children into conformity with our expectations by drugging them with Ritalin, Concerta, and Adderall, when we really need to foster their independence and courage.

We can hope to realize that it's a disservice to ourselves and to our children to mute the spirit of our more vigorous and rambunctious girls and boys by diagnosing and drugging them.

We can hope to place less emphasis on growing up to be well rounded and to put more emphasis on growing up to be creative and daring, and even rugged and tough when necessary.

We need to reaffirm the truth taught by most religions—including Judaism, Christianity, and Islam—that human life is fragile, that the world is dangerous, and that each individual must embrace life with love, courage, and unflinching ethics and principles. Instead of using diagnoses like ADHD and drugs like Ritalin and Adderall to smother our children's spirits, we need to admire their special energy and spunk, and to find ways to guide them in more positive directions.

The times are still too raw to be sure of our new perspectives. We remain as yet too close to the dreadful events that began to unfold on September 11. But we should not shirk the task of asking ourselves the meaning of these events in regard to our expectations of our children. The future is already testing our youth as many of them go to war and as others prepare to deal with grave uncertainties. If it is not already doing so, the future will soon be testing our younger children as well.

In *Reclaiming Our Children* (2000a), I warned that the psychiatric approach is crushing our "warrior children"—our youngsters with the most critical intelligence and the most determination to stand up for what they believe, even in the face of threat and danger. I warned that we were producing future generations that would live in fear of being different and always seek to placate and please. It's now more apparent than ever that those in future generations will require a measure of independence in thought and action that's incompatible with threatening to diagnose and drug them as children when they step out of line, challenge us, or fail to meet our expectations.

If we are inspired to place more emphasis on promoting courage and determination in our children, then it will be one more of those gifts that has come unexpectedly from the tragic events of recent times.

Notes

Introduction

1. Focalin is a new product from Novartis. Many pharmacological agents come in slightly different forms called isomers. Isomers that are mirror images of each other are referred to as left- and right-handed. Focalin consists of the right-handed version of methylphenidate (dexmethylphenidate). It is said to be more potent and hence to require lower doses. However, there is no reason to believe that the isomer will cause fewer adverse effects. In addition, as this book will describe, the active or "therapeutic" impact of a stimulant drug is actually one of its most harmful effects.

Chapter 2: A Child's Journey Through Psychiatric Diagnoses and Drugs

1. The story of Alec is a composite made up from several different stories. I've combined stories to disguise any one particular child's identity, but Alec sounds so much like so many of my patients that some parents may be sure I'm talking about their child.

2. Also see Chapter 10 of this book. For a more detailed discussion of tardive dyskinesia, see Breggin (1997a). For an introduction, see Breggin and Cohen (1999). A Task Force Report on tardive dyskinesia by the American Psychiatric Association (1980) estimated that at least 10–20 percent of patients exposed relatively short-term (a year or more) will develop tardive dyskinesia and that 40 percent of longer-term patients will develop it. The American Psychiatric Association's (2000) *DSM-IV-TR* suggests a rate of 3–5 percent per year cumulative. The best studies, reviewed in Breggin (1997a), reveal a cumulative rate of 5–8 percent per year. These rates have been established in adults. However, the rates are high in children as well. Tardive dyskinesia in children is likely to be even more disabling, often involving distortions of the trunk, posture, and walking. See Breggin (1997a) for details. Whatever rate one decides on, the risk is so extraordinary that few if any parents would give their children this kind of drug if they knew the risk, and few adults would take these drugs if they were fully informed of the

dangers. Tardive dyskinesia usually but not always requires three months of exposure to the drugs before it appears. In children, it may take less time. All antipsychotics, including newer ones like Risperdal, Zyprexa, and Seroquel, are required by the FDA to carry a class warning for tardive dyskinesia. This class warning was mandated after my 1983 book generated widespread publicity including a news story by Dan Rather that exposed the dangers of tardive dyskinesia. My 1983 book was among the very first, if not the first, to warn about the extent of the danger of tardive dyskinesia in children.

3. Rosebush and Mazurek (1999).

4. Tardive dyskinesia can afflict any voluntary muscle. The voluntary muscles are under conscious control, in contrast to the muscles of the digestive organs, heart, and other bodily functions that are not usually under conscious control.

Chapter 3: Of Cages and Creativity—How Stimulants Work

1. In *Talking Back to Ritalin* (rev. ed., 2001a) and in my peer-reviewed scientific publications (Breggin, 1999a, 1999b, 1999c), I cite numerous relevant animal studies that demonstrate the crushing of spontaneous behavior and the enforcement of asocial, stereotypical, or compulsive behavior in animals exposed to routine doses of stimulants. A few examples include Castner et al. (2000); Castner and Goldman-Rakic (1999); Costall and Naylor (1974); Bell et al., (1982); Koek and Colpaert (1993); Arakawa (1994); Sams-Dodd and Newman (1997); Conti et al. (1997); Melega et al. (1997a). The recent stimulant studies of rhesus monkeys are Castner et al. (2000) and especially Castner and Goldman-Rakic (1999). These studies confirm that Ritalin and amphetamine, and indeed cocaine, have similar effects.

2. Castner et al. (2000) and Castner and Goldman-Rakic (1999). The latter has the most detailed descriptions.

3. Later chapters will provide additional scientific basis for the observation I am making connecting the effects on animals with those seen in children.

4. Table 3.1 was originally prepared for my presentation on adverse drug effects to the November 1998 Consensus Development Conference on the Diagnosis and Treatment of Attention Deficit Hyperactivity Disorder (Breggin, 1998a) and has appeared in several of my peer-reviewed papers.

5. See studies of overfocusing in stimulated treated children by Dyme et al. (1982) and Solanto and Wender (1989). Borcherding et al. (1990) describe high rates of compulsive behavior in children taking stimulants. All of these issues will be dealt with at greater length in this book.

Chapter 4: How Stimulants Cause Psychiatric Disorders

1. Reviewed in more detail in Breggin (1999a, 1999c, 2001a). These hundreds of reports were made spontaneously to the FDA, mostly by physicians

and hospital pharmacists who went to the trouble to fill out the appropriate forms. Most of these busy professionals would not go to this trouble if they did not believe that the drug probably caused the harmful effect. Each individual report may or may not prove a direct causal relationship between the drug and the bad outcome, but the pattern is clear: Stimulants commonly cause severe emotional disturbances in children.

2. Swanson et al. (1992).

3. Whalen and Henker (1997).

4. From Maxmen and Ward (1995, p. 366).

5. Breggin (1999b, 1999c).

6. Data for the estimate are presented in Breggin (1999c, p. 10).

7. Efron et al. (1997). This was a double-blind, crossover study.

8. Mayes et al. (1994).

9. Because it is a new drug, the 2002 Adderall XR label did not appear in the 2002 *Physicians' Desk Reference* and was therefore taken off the company web site.

10. Cherland and Fitzpatrick (1999). At one point the authors give the figure of 9 children out of 98 developing "psychotic symptoms" (p. 812), consistent with the 9 cases listed in their Table 1, entitled "Children with Psychotic Effects," for a rate of 9 percent. At another time they refer to a rate of 6 percent for "psychotic side effects" (also p. 812) and an 11.7 percent rate for "mood-only symptoms or mood-congruent psychotic symptoms while being treated with MPH [methylphenidate] (11.7%)." "Mood only" and "mood congruent" refer to emotional symptoms such as mania and depression with and without psychotic symptoms such as hallucinations. However these data are read, it is clear that a sizable portion (probably in the range of 10 percent or more) of the children developed serious psychotic symptoms attributable to the drugs.

11. Arnold and Jensen (1995, p. 2307).

12. Borcherding et al. (1990).

13. Solanto and Wender (1989).

Chapter 5: How Stimulants Harm the Child's Brain

1. Vastag (2001).

2. Wang et al. (1994). The dose was 0.5 mg/kg intravenously. Oral doses would produce a similar but perhaps less acute effect. The brain scan was the PET, or Positron Emission Tomography. For a lengthier review of the literature confirming brain dysfunction and damage from stimulant drugs, see Breggin (1999a, 1999b, 1999c, 2001a).

3. Porrino and Lucignani (1987).

4. For how drug companies control research, see my 1991 book, *Toxic Psychiatry*, as well as my other books (e.g., Breggin 1997a, 2001a). The problem has been much more broadly recognized since then and has even

been raised by editorials and commentaries in the most prestigious medical and scientific journals; for example, see Angell et al. (2000), Bodenheimer (2000), Morton (2000), and Thompson (1993).

5. Breggin (1999a, 1999b, 1999c).

6. Robinson and Kolb (1997).

7. Melega et al. (1997b).

8. Melega et al. (1997a).

9. Sonsalla et al. (1996) found dopaminergic cell loss of 40–50 percent in the substantia nigra. Battaglia et al. (1987) found "long-lasting neurotoxic effects with respect to both the functional and structural integrity of serotonergic neurons in the brain" (p. 911).

10. Dougherty et al. (1999).

11. Vastag (2001).

12. The quote is taken from the University of Buffalo (2001) web site press release.

13. Ellinwood and Tong (1996).

14. Jaffe (1995). Neuronal loss indicates cell death; microhemorrhages are small areas of bleeding inside the brain.

15. In Castner et al. (2000), rhesus monkeys were given twice-daily injections of amphetamine or placebo for six weeks with weekends off. The dose rose from 0.1 mg/kg to 1.0 mg/kg. In another study, Caster and Goldman-Rakic (1999), the animals were given the regimen over twelve weeks. The single challenge dose given to determine brain sensitization to the drug was only 0.4 mg/kg. Typical treatment doses for ADHD are in the range of 0.5 mg/kg, but it is not unheard of for doctors to prescribe in excess of 1.0 mg/kg. At 1 mg/kg, a child weighing 45.5 kg (100 pounds) would receive 45.5 mg per day of stimulant. The 2001 label for Adderall states: "Only in rare cases will it be necessary to exceed a total of 40 mg per day" for ADHD. This indicates that the FDA-approved upper range (which is too often exceeded in clinical practice) approximates the highest dose briefly given to the animals for a few days at the end of the treatment period. Furthermore, clinical treatment usually goes on for many months and years, rather than 6–12 weeks. Clinical treatment also often involves other potentially toxic drugs. In short, monkeys developed long-term sensitization to amphetamine at doses in the clinical range over very short exposure times.

16. Castner et al. (2000, p. 10, bottom of first column).

17. Nasrallah et al. (1986).

18. Reviewed in Breggin (2001a).

19. Castellanos et al. (1998) and Giedd et al. (1994) are two of the studies cited by Swanson and others to show that ADHD is biological when they should be cited to show that stimulant drugs permanently damage the brains of children. While these studies often obscure the fact that the children were taking drugs at the time of or shortly before the brain scans, Swanson acknowledged at the conference that none of them studied children with

no drug-exposure history. I pointed out to the conference that Swanson and the other researchers were behaving unethically when they failed to announce up front that the children had been exposed to psychoactive substances. For a more detailed review of these studies, see Breggin (2001a).

20. Ellison et al. (1996, p. 121).

21. The connection was first made by my research assistant, Ian Goddard, when he read Ellison et al. (1996).

Chapter 6: How Stimulants Harm the Child's Body

1. Safer, Allan, and Barr (1975).

2. Reviewed in Breggin (2001a, pp. 51–54).

3. Jacobvitz et al. (1990).

4. Yudofsky et al. (1991).

5. Spencer et al. (1996).

6. Breggin (1999a and 1999c). From 1985 to March 3, 1997, there were 2,821 reports of adverse Ritalin effects sent to the FDA. Most of the reports were made by doctors and pharmacists.

7. Karch (1996); Henderson and Fischer (1994); Ishiguro and Morgan (1997).

8. Brown and Sexton (1988).

9. Buxton and McConachie (2001).

10. Trugman (1988).

11. Schteinschnaider et al. (2000).

12. Epstein (2000).

13. As with most of the material in this chapter, I have covered this subject in much greater detail in Breggin (1997a, 1999a, 1999c).

14. Firestone et al. (1998).

15. Borcherding et al. (1990).

16. Lipkin et al. (1994).

17. Varley et al. (2001). The authors wonder if the tics developed spontaneously or if they were caused by the drugs; but they admit that a spontaneous rate of 8 percent for tics in children without drugs is high. In fact, considering that the observations were made over a limited period of treatment, it's absurd to think that there would be an 8-percent rate of spontaneously developing tics in drug-free children. Also, the rates were higher in the younger children, confirming they were drug-induced in the more vulnerable population.

18. Breggin (1999a and 1999c).

19. Described in the 2001 Ritalin label as "hypersensitivity (including skin rash, urticaria, fever, arthralgias, exfoliative dermatitis, erythema multiforme with histological findings of necrotizing vasculitis, and thrombocytopenic purpura). . . ." A number of these are as dreadful as they sound, including excruciating pain and possible death. Some of them probably reflect an autoimmune response. Thrombocytopenic purpura is caused by a loss of

platelets that circulate in the blood and are necessary for clotting. The purpura refers to the development of visible bleeding into the skin (can look like bruises) when the platelets are decreased.

20. The Adderall XR label was mailed as an addendum to the 2001 *Physicians' Desk Reference* and appears in the 2002 edition.

21. National Toxicology Program (1995, p. 11). Discussed in greater detail with citations in Breggin (2001a, p. 42).

22. I have written about neuroleptic malignant syndrome (NMS) in Breggin (1990, 1993).

23. Firestone et al. (1998).

Chapter 7: How Stimulants Cause Withdrawal, Addiction, and Abuse

1. The same warning appears at the beginning of the Adderall XR label, but somehow the FDA allowed the manufacturer to leave off the damning conclusion "and must be avoided."

2. Drug Enforcement Administration (DEA) (1993, 1995a, 1995b, 1995c, 1996). International Narcotics Control Board (INCB) (1995, 1997).

3. Feussner (1998).

4. Drug Enforcement Administration (1995c).

5. International Narcotics Control Board (INCB) (1995, 1997).

6. Riordan and Matyas (1994) is the legal brief for CHADD's attempt to influence the DEA to drop Ritalin from Schedule II. CHADD claimed that Ritalin was not addictive or subject to abuse. As noted in the text, I have written about CHADD, Novartis, and the politics and economics of ADHD in some depth in *Talking Back to Ritalin* (rev. ed., 2001a).

7. The DEA's heavily documented response to CHADD can be found in Drug Enforcement Administration (1995c) and Feussner (1998).

8. Volkow et al. (1995). I have reviewed the science behind these observations in some depth in *Talking Back to Ritalin* (rev. ed., 2001a) and in my professional articles (e.g., Breggin, 1999a, 1999b, 1999c). For general discussions of stimulant addiction by a professional whose work has spanned decades, see Ellinwood and Cohen (1972) and Ellinwood and Tong (1996).

9. *Archives of General Psychiatry* (June 1995, p. 422).

10. Lambert (1998) and Lambert and Hartsough (1998).

11. Rapoport et al. (1978). The dose was 0.5 mg/kg amphetamine. The study was published in *Science*, one of the most prestigious journals in the world, but seemingly had no impact on prescription practices.

Chapter 9: Do Stimulants Really Help with "ADHD"?

1. Popper and Steingard (1994).

2. Richters et al. (1995).

3. Whalen and Henker (1997).

4. Swanson (circa 1993).

5. Emphasis added.

6. Gillberg et al. (1997).

7. Breggin (2000e, 2000f, 2001c).

Chapter 10: Do Antidepressants and Other Drugs Help with "ADHD"?

1. I discuss the stimulating effects of selective serotonin reuptake inhibitors (SSRIs) in detail in *Talking Back to Prozac* (with Ginger Breggin, 1994), *Brain-Disabling Treatments in Psychiatry* (1997a) and *The Antidepressant Fact Book* (2001b). All of the material in this section is covered in depth in those books.

2. Hence they are classified as SSRIs.

3. Emslie et al. (1997). The researchers buried the data so that it has to be picked out of the section on reasons for dropouts.

4. Jain et al. (1992).

5. I confirmed that Eric Harris had a "therapeutic level" of Luvox in his blood at autopsy from records I obtained from the FDA under the Freedom of Information Act. See Breggin (2000a and 2002, in press).

6. Marangell et al. (1999, p. 1038).

7. Garland and Baerg (2001).

8. For Prozac animal studies, see Wegerer et al. (1999) and Norrholm and Ouimet (2000). For the Paxil children study, see Gilbert et al. (2000).

9. For more details about antipsychotic drugs, including rates for tardive dyskinesia and neuroleptic malignant syndrome, see my medical book *Brain-Disabling Treatments in Psychiatry* (1997a), or my more popular book *Your Drug May Be Your Problem* (with David Cohen, 1999).

10. Addonizio et al. (1986). See Breggin (1997a) for details.

11. For a description of TD and the citation of these conservative rates, see American Psychiatric Association (2000).

12. See Rosebush and Mazurek (1999).

Chapter 11: Do "Alternative Treatments" Help with "ADHD"?

1. Scientific issues related to alternatives, including the hypoglycemia theory, are reviewed in my book *Talking Back to Ritalin* (rev. ed., 2001a).

Chapter 12: The Ultimate Source of Misinformation

1. I have written about the control of information in psychiatry in many books, starting with *Toxic Psychiatry* (1991) and continuing through several others (e.g., Breggin 1997a; Breggin and Breggin, 1994 and 1998). *Talking Back to Ritalin* (rev. ed., 2001a) covers the stimulant/ADHD industry in the most detail.

2. Psychiatric adverse effects are usually found in a section entitled "Adverse Effects" with a subtitle of "Central Nervous System."

3. Information on the length of the trial is buried in the text in the following observation: "Adverse events reported in a 3-week clinical trial of

pediatric patients treated with ADDERALL XR™ or placebo are presented in the table below." To add to the confusion, the table is not "below" but above. (There's only one table in the label.) A doctor reading through this label for information before prescribing would be hard pressed to figure out that the only table for adverse events in the label was based on a study of only three weeks in length. It takes a very careful study of the label with a trained critical eye to disentangle this information. It is astonishing that the FDA let Shire US Inc. get away with using such a short trial and then with failing to mention its length in the table itself.

4. Sabshin (1992) wrote the letter on behalf of the American Psychiatric Association in response to my earlier letter (Breggin, 1992b).

5. Angell et al. (2000); Bodenheimer (2000).

Chapter 13: The Real Nature of "ADHD"

1. For my most recent analysis of antidepressant-induced harm to the brain, see *The Antidepressant Fact Book* (2001b).

2. Joseph (2000b).

3. In *Talking Back to Ritalin* (rev. ed., 2001a), I devoted an entire chapter to potential causes for ADHD-like behavior.

4. My assistant, Ian Goddard, made this keen observation.

5. Some neurological disorders will wax and wane; that is, they will appear worse at some times and better at others. Often they will temporarily improve if the person is more relaxed and worsen if the person is more distressed. However, they will rarely disappear in any particular setting for any length of time. Furthermore, the individual would be unable to completely transcend the disorder to function on an especially high level, as many supposedly ADHD children will do when involved with activities that they love such as computer or sports activities.

Chapter 14: The Real Nature of "Learning Disorders"

1. For additional critiques of learning disabilities, see Coles (1987) and Valentine (1988).

2. I propose and discuss the concept of critical intelligence in *Reclaiming Our Children* (2000a).

3. Gardner (1993).

Chapter 15: Why "ADHD" Should Not Be Considered a Disability

1. See Breggin and Breggin (1998), *The War Against Children of Color*.

Chapter 16: How to Provide Guidance in the Family

1. Several books on how to help children have been written by active opponents of the concept of ADHD and stimulants. Some of these authors are members of the organization that I founded thirty-plus years ago, the International Center for the Study of Psychiatry and Psychology (for example,

Stein, 1999, 2001; Valentine, 1987, 1988; Oas, 2001; Glasser, 1998). Levine (2001) provides a critique and some suggestions. In addition, there are many generic, good books on child rearing that can be found on the bookshelves of stores, including the granddaddy of them all (Gordon, 1970). I have written several chapters on parenting and teaching in *Talking Back to Ritalin* (rev. ed., 2001a) and address becoming a helping person in *The Heart of Being Helpful* (1997b).

2. For example, Gordon (1970), Ginott (1969), and Covey (1997).

3. I discuss the moral qualities of children in *Beyond Conflict* (1992a).

Chapter 19: When the School Says Your Child Has a Problem

1. See my book *Reclaiming Our Children* (2000a) for a discussion of peer abuse and many other subjects touched on in this chapter.

2. See my book *Reclaiming Our Children* (2000a) for a discussion of alternatives, from private schools to home schooling.

Chapter 20: Getting Worse Before It Gets Better

1. Zernike and Petersen (2001).

2. The drug company that makes Metadate, Celltech Pharmaceuticals, is based in Great Britain. A 1971 international treaty bans direct advertising of Schedule II drugs because they are the most addictive used in medicine. However, there are no federal laws to prohibit the direct advertising of these substances to the consumer. Nonetheless, a DEA official states, "We have had a 30-year agreement with the pharmaceutical industry not to advertise controlled substances" (quoted in Zernike and Petersen [2001]). The DEA has also said that the McNeil ads for Concerta on TV break the spirit if not the letter of the law. Unfortunately, the U.S. Food and Drug Administration (FDA) has shown virtually no concern about the dangers of these drugs and has approved the more aggressive advertising.

3. The 4–6 million figure is my own estimate, up from the 4–5 million estimate I made in *Talking Back to Ritalin* (rev. ed., 2001a). The 4–6 million estimate was also adopted in an August report in the *Journal of the American Medical Association* (Vastag, 2001).

4. The study data is taken from Marshall (2000). The figure of 20% is taken from an editorial in *USA Today* (2000) that cites additional study data.

5. Breggin, *Talking Back to Ritalin* (rev. ed., 2001a).

Bibliography

Addonizio, G., Susman, V., and Roth, S. (1986). Symptoms of neuroleptic malignant syndrome in 82 consecutive inpatients. *American Journal of Psychiatry* 143:1587–1590.

American Psychiatric Association. (1980). *Task Force Report 18: Tardive Dyskinesia*. Washington, D.C.: American Psychiatric Association.

American Psychiatric Association. (1994). *Diagnostic and Statistical Manual of Mental Disorders, IV (DSM-IV)*. Washington, D.C.: American Psychiatric Association.

American Psychiatric Association. (2000). *Diagnostic and Statistical Manual of Mental Disorders, IV*, rev. text *(DSM-IV-TR)*. Washington, D.C.: American Psychiatric Association.

Angell, M., Utiger, R., and Wood, A. (2000, February 24). Disclosure of authors' conflict of interest: A follow-up. *New England Journal of Medicine* 342:586–587.

Arakawa, O. (1994). Effects of methamphetamine and methylphenidate on single and paired rat open-field behaviors. *Physiology and Behavior* 55:441–446.

Archives of General Psychiatry. (1995, June). Editorial. 52:422–423.

Arnold, L. E., and Jensen, P. S. (1995). Attention-deficit disorders. In H. I. Kaplan and B. Sadock, eds., *Comprehensive Textbook of Psychiatry*, 4th ed., pp. 2295–2310. Baltimore: Williams and Wilkins.

Battaglia, G., Yeh, S., O'Hearn, E., Molliver, M., Kuhar, M., and De Souza, E. (1987). 3,4-methylenedioxymethamphetamine and 3,4-methylenedioxyamphetamine destroy serotonin terminals in rat brain. *Journal of Pharmacology and Experimental Therapeutics* 242:911–916.

Bell, R. D., Alexander, G. M., Schwartzman, R. J., and Yu, J. (1982). The methylphenidate-induced stereotypy in the awake rat: Local cerebral metabolism. *Neurology* 32:377–381.

Bodenheimer, T. (2000, May 18). Uneasy alliance: Clinical investigators and the pharmaceutical industry. *New England Journal of Medicine* 342:1539–1544.

Borcherding, B. V., Keysor, C. S., Rapoport, J. L., Elia, J., and Amass, J. (1990). Motor/vocal tics and compulsive behaviors on stimulant drugs: Is there a common vulnerability? *Psychiatric Research* 33:83–94.

Breggin, P. (1983). *Psychiatric Drugs: Hazards to the Brain*. New York: Springer Publishing Company.

Breggin, P. (1990). Brain damage, dementia and persistent cognitive dysfunction associated with neuroleptic drugs: Evidence, etiology, implications. *Journal of Mind and Behavior* 11:425–464.

Breggin, P. (1991). *Toxic Psychiatry: Why Therapy, Empathy and Love Must Replace the Drugs, Electroshock and Biochemical Theories of the "New Psychiatry."* New York: HarperCollins.

Breggin, P. (1992a). *Beyond Conflict: From Self-Help and Psychotherapy to Peacemaking.* New York: St. Martin's Press.

Breggin, P. (1992b, February 11). Letter. The president's sleeping pill and its maker. *New York Times.*

Breggin, P. (1993). Parallels between neuroleptic effects and lethargic encephalitis: The production of dyskinesias and cognitive disorders. *Brain and Cognition* 23:8–27.

Breggin, P. (1997a). *Brain-Disabling Treatments in Psychiatry: Drugs, Electroshock and the Role of the FDA.* New York: Springer Publishing Company.

Breggin, P. (1997b). *The Heart of Being Helpful: Empathy and the Creation of a Healing Presence.* New York: Springer Publishing Company.

Breggin, P. (1997c). Psychotherapy in emotional crises without resort to psychiatric medication. *Humanistic Psychologist* 25:2–14.

Breggin, P. (1998a). Risks and mechanism of action of stimulants. *Program and Abstracts*, pp. 105–120. NIH Consensus Development Conference on the Diagnosis and Treatment of Attention Deficit Hyperactivity Disorder. November 16–18, 1998, William H. Natcher Conference Center, National Institutes of Health, Bethesda, MD.

Breggin, P. (1998b). Data compiled and analyzed by the author from Food and Drug Administration (1997).

Breggin, P. (1998c). Analysis of adverse behavioral effects of benzodiazepines with a discussion of drawing scientific conclusions from the FDA's Spontaneous Reporting System. *Journal of Mind and Behavior* 19:21–50.

Breggin, P. (1998d). Risks and mechanism of action of stimulants. *NIH Consensus Development Conference Program and Abstracts: Diagnosis and Treatment of Attention Deficit Hyperactivity Disorder*, pp. 105–120. Rockville, MD: National Institutes of Health.

Breggin, P. (1999a). Psychostimulants in the treatment of children diagnosed with ADHD: Part I: Acute risks and psychological effects. *Ethical Human Sciences and Services* 1:13–33.

Breggin, P. (1999b). Psychostimulants in the treatment of children diagnosed with ADHD: Part II: Adverse effects on brain and behavior. *Ethical Human Sciences and Services* 1:213–241.

Breggin, P. (1999c). Psychostimulants in the treatment of children diagnosed with ADHD: Risks and mechanism of action. *International Journal of Risk and Safety in Medicine* 12:3–35. Simultaneously published in two parts by Springer Publishing Company, in *Ethical Human Sciences and Services* (Breggin 1999a and b).

Breggin, P. (2000a). *Reclaiming Our Children: A Healing Solution for a Nation in Crisis.* Cambridge: Perseus Publishing.

Breggin, P. (2000b, February 28). Don't let "experts" parent your children. *USA Today*.

Breggin, P. (2000c). What psychologists and psychotherapists need to know about ADHD and stimulants. *Changes: An International Journal of Psychology and Psychotherapy* 18 (Spring):13–23.

Breggin, P. (2000d, September 29). Testimony concerning behavioral drug use in the schools before the U.S. House of Representatives Committee on Education and the Workforce, Subcommittee on Oversight and Investigations, Washington, D.C. Text of Breggin's formal submission to the committee available at www.breggin.com. See U.S. House of Representatives, 2000, for how to purchase C-Span film of entire hearing.

Breggin, P. (2000e). The NIMH multimodal study of treatment for attention-deficit/hyperactivity disorder: A critical analysis. *International Journal of Risk and Safety in Medicine* 13:15–22.

Breggin, P. (2000f). A critical analysis of the NIMH multimodal treatment study for Attention-Deficit Hyperactivity Disorder (the MTA study). *Ethical Human Sciences and Services* 2:63–72.

Breggin, P. (2001a). *Talking Back to Ritalin: What Doctors Aren't Telling You About Stimulants for Children*, rev. ed. Cambridge: Perseus Publishing.

Breggin, P. (2001b). *The Antidepressant Fact Book: What Your Doctor Won't Tell You About Prozac, Zoloft, Paxil, Celexa, and Luvox*. Cambridge: Perseus Publishing.

Breggin, P. (2001c). Letter. MTA study [NIMH clinical trials on stimulants for ADHD] has flaws. *Archives of General Psychiatry* 58:1184.

Breggin, P. (2002, in press). Fluvoxamine as a cause of stimulation, mania, and aggression with a critical analysis of the FDA-approved label. *International Journal of Risk and Safety in Medicine*.

Breggin, P., and Breggin, G. (1994). *Talking Back to Prozac: What Doctors Aren't Telling You About Today's Most Controversial Drug*. New York: St. Martin's Press.

Breggin, P., and Breggin, G. (1998). *The War Against Children of Color: Psychiatry Targets Inner-City Youth*. Monroe, ME: Common Courage Press.

Breggin, P., Breggin, G., and Bemak, F. (2002). *Dimensions of Empathic Therapy*. New York: Springer Publishing Company.

Breggin, P., and Cohen, D. (1999). *Your Drug May Be Your Problem: How and Why to Stop Taking Psychiatric Medications*. Cambridge: Perseus Publishing.

Breggin, P., and Stern, E. M., eds. (1996). *Psychosocial Approaches to Deeply Disturbed Persons*. New York: Haworth Press.

Brown, R. T., and Sexton, S. B. (1988). A controlled trial of methylphenidate in black adolescents. *Clinical Pediatrics* 27:74–81.

Brown, W. A., and William, B. W. (1976). Methylphenidate increases serum growth hormone concentrations. *Journal of Clinical Endocrinology and Metabolism* 43:937–938.

Buxton, N., and McConachie, N. (2001). Amphetamine abuse and intracranial haemorrhage. *Journal of the Royal Society of Medicine* 93:472–477.

Castellanos, F. X., Giedd, J. N., Elia, J., Marsh, W. L., Ritchie, G. F., Hamburger, S. D., and Rapoport, J. L. (1997). Controlled stimulant treatment of ADHD and Comorbid Tourette's syndrome: Effects of stimulant and dose. *Journal of the American Academy of Child and Adolescent Psychiatry* 36:589–596.

Castellanos, F. X., Giedd, J. N., Marsh, W. L., Hamburger, S. D., Vaituzis, A. C., Dickstein, D. P., Sarfatti, S. E., Vauss, Y. C., Snell, J. W., Lange, N., Kaysen, D., Krain, A. L., Ritchie, G. F., Rajapakse, J. C., and Rapoport, J. L. (1998). Quantitative brain magnetic resonance imaging in attention-deficit hyperactivity disorder. *Archives of General Psychiatry* 53:607–616.

Castner, S., Al-Tikriti, M., Baldwin, R., Seibyl, J., Innis, R., and Goldman-Rakic, P. (2000). Behavioral changes and [123]IBZM equilibrium SPECT measurement of amphetamine-induced dopamine release in rhesus monkeys exposed to subchronic amphetamine. *Neuropsychopharmacology* 22:4–13.

Castner, S., and Goldman-Rakic, P. (1999). Long-lasting psychotomimetic consequences of repeated low-dose amphetamine exposure in rhesus monkeys. *Neuropsychopharmacology* 20:10–28.

Cherland, E., and Fitzpatrick, R. (1999). Psychotic side effects of psychostimulants: A 5-year review. *Canadian Journal of Psychiatry* 44:811–813.

Coles, G. (1987). *The Learning Mystique: A Critical Look at "Learning Disabilities."* New York: Pantheon Books.

Conti, L. H., Segal, D. S., and Kuczenski, R. (1997). Maintenance of amphetamine-induced stereotypy and locomotion requires ongoing dopamine receptor activation. *Psychopharmacology* 130:183–188.

Costall, B., and Naylor, R. J. (1974). The involvement of dopaminergic systems with the stereotyped behavior patterns induced by methylphenidate. *Journal of Pharmacy and Pharmacology* 26:30–33.

Covey, S. (1997). *The 7 Habits of Highly Effective Families.* New York: Golden Books.

Dougherty, D., Bonab, A., Spencer, T., Rauch, S., Madras, B., and Fischman, A. (1999, December 18/25). Dopamine transporter density in patients with attention deficit disorder. *Lancet* 354:2132–2133.

Drug Enforcement Administration (DEA). (1993, October 7). Public Affairs press release concerning Aggregate Production Quota for methylphenidate. Washington, D.C.: Public Affairs Section, DEA, U.S. Department of Justice.

Drug Enforcement Administration (DEA). (1995a, October 20). Methylphenidate: DEA press release [attached to DEA, 1995b]. Washington, D.C.: Drug and Chemical Evaluation Section, Office of Diversion Control, DEA, U.S. Department of Justice.

Drug Enforcement Administration (DEA). (1995b, October). Methylphenidate (a background paper). Washington, D.C.: Drug and Chemical Evaluation Section, Office of Diversion Control, DEA, U.S. Department of Justice.

Drug Enforcement Administration (DEA). (1995c, August 7). Response to CHADD petition concerning Ritalin. Washington, D.C.: DEA, U.S. Department of Justice.

Drug Enforcement Administration (DEA). (1996, December 10–12). Conference report: Stimulant use in the treatment of ADHD. Washington, D.C.: DEA, U.S. Department of Justice.

Dulcan, M. (1994). Treatment of children and adolescents. In R. Hales, Yudofsky, S. and Talbott, J. (eds.), *The American Psychiatric Press Textbook of Psychiatry* (2nd ed.), pp. 1209–1250. Washington; D.C.: American Psychiatric Press.

Dyme, I. Z., Sahakian, B. J., Golinko, B. E., and Rabe, E. F. (1982). Perseveration induced by methylphenidate in children: Preliminary findings. *Progress in Neuro-Psychopharmacology and Biological Psychiatry* 6:269–273.

Efron, D., Jarman, F. C., and Barker, M. J. (1997). Side effects of methylphenidate and dexamphetamine in children with attention deficit hyperactivity disorder: A double-blind, crossover trial. *Pediatrics* 100:662–666.

Ellinwood, E. H., and Cohen, S. (1972). *Current Concepts of Amphetamine Abuse*. Rockville, MD: National Institute of Mental Health. DHEW Publication No. (HSM) 72-9085.

Ellinwood, E. H., and Tong, H. L. (1996). Central nervous system stimulants and anorectic agents. In M.N.G. Dukes, ed., *Meyler's Side Effects of Drugs: An Encyclopedia of Adverse Reactions and Interactions,* 13th ed., pp. 1–30. New York: Elsevier.

Ellison, G., Irwin, S., Keys, A., Noguchi, K., and Sulur, G. (1996). The neurotoxic effects of continuous cocaine and amphetamine in habenula: Implications for the substrates of psychosis. *NIDA Research Monographs* 163:117–195.

Emslie, G. J., Rush, A. J., Weinberg, W. A., Kowatch, R. A., Hughes, C. W., Carmody, T., and Rintelmann, J. (1997). A double-blind, randomized, placebo-controlled trial of fluoxetine in children and adolescents with depression. *Archives of General Psychiatry* 54:1031–1037.

Epstein, K. (2000, May 2). Ephedra: Behind the headlines. *Washington Post, Health* magazine.

Feussner, G. (1998). Diversion, trafficking, and abuse of methylphenidate. *NIH Consensus Development Conference Program and Abstracts: Diagnosis and Treatment of Attention Deficit Hyperactivity Disorder,* pp. 201–204. Rockville, MD: National Institutes of Health.

Fialkov, J., and Hasley, S. (1984). Psychotropic drug effects contributing to psychiatric hospitalization of children: A preliminary study. *Developmental and Behavioral Pediatrics* 5:325–330.

Firestone, P., Musten, L. M., Pisterman, S., Mercer, J., and Bennett, S. (1998). Short-term side effects of stimulant medications in preschool children with attention-deficit/hyperactivity disorder: A double-blind placebo-controlled study. *Journal of Child and Adolescent Psychopharmacology* 8:13–25.

Food and Drug Administration (FDA). (1997, March). Spontaneous Reporting System (SRS) data for methylphenidate: 1985 through March 3, 1997. Rockville, MD. Obtained through Freedom of Information Act (FOIA).

Gardner, H. (1993). *Multiple Intelligences: The Theory in Practice*. New York: Basic Books.

Garland, E., and Baerg, E. (2001). Amotivational syndrome associated with selective serotonin reuptake inhibitors in children and adolescents. *Journal of Child and Adolescent Psychopharmacology* 11:181–186.

Giedd, J., Castellanos, F., Casey, B., Kozuch, P., King, A., Hamburger, S. D., and Rapoport, J. L. (1994). Quantitative morphology of the corpus callosum in attention deficit hyperactivity disorder. *American Journal of Psychiatry* 151:665–669.

Gilbert, A., Moore, G., Keshavan, M., Paulson, L., Narula, V., Mac Master, P., Stewart, C., and Rosenberg, D. (2000). Decreased thalamic volumes of pediatric patients with obsessive-compulsive disorder who are taking paroxetine. *Archives of General Psychiatry* 57:449–456.

Gillberg, C., Melander, H., von Knorring, A.-L., Janols, L.-O., Thernlund, G., Hagglof, B., Eidevall-Wallin, L., Gustafsson, P., and Kopp S. (1997). Long-term stimulant treatment of children with attention-deficit hyperactivity disorder symptoms: A randomized, double-blind, placebo-controlled trial. *Archives of General Psychiatry* 54:857–864.

Ginott, H. (1969). *Between Parent and Child.* New York: Avon.

Glasser, W. (1998). *Choice Theory.* New York: HarperCollins.

Gordon, T. (1970). *P.E.T.: Parent Effectiveness Training.* New York: Peter H. Wyden.

Henderson, T. A., and Fischer, V. W. (1994). Effects of methylphenidate (Ritalin) on mammalian myocardial ultrastructure. *American Journal of Cardiovascular Pathology* 5:68–78.

Hynd, G. W., Semrud-Clikeman, M., Lorys, A. R., Novey, E. S., Eliopulos, D., and Lyytinen, H. (1991). Corpus callosum morphology in attention deficit-hyperactivity disorder: Morphometric analysis on MRI. *Journal of Learning Disabilities* 24:141–145.

International Narcotics Control Board (INCB). (1995, February 28). Dramatic increase in methylphenidate consumption in U.S.: Marketing methods questioned. *INCB Annual Report 1995: Background Note No. 2.* Vienna, Austria: Author.

International Narcotics Control Board (INCB). (1997, March 4). INCB sees continuing risk in stimulant prescribed for children. *INCB Annual Report: Background Note No. 4.* Vienna, Austria: Author.

Ishiguro, Y., and Morgan, J. P. (1997). Biphasic inotropic effects of methamphetamine and methylphenidate on ferret papillary muscles. *Journal of Cardiovascular Pharmacology* 30:744–749.

Jacobvitz, D., Sroufe, L. A., Stewart, M., and Leffert, N. (1990). Treatment of attentional and hyperactivity problems in children with sympathomimetic drugs: A comprehensive review. *Journal of the American Academy of Child and Adolescent Psychiatry* 29:677–688.

Jaffe, J. (1995). Amphetamine (or amphetaminelike)-related disorders. In H. Kaplan and B. Sadock, eds., *Comprehensive Textbook of Psychiatry,* vol. 6, pp. 791–799. Baltimore: Williams and Wilkins.

Jain, J., Birmaher, B., Garcia, M., Al-Shabbout, M., and Ryan, N. (1992). Fluoxetine in children and adolescents with mood disorders: A chart review of efficacy and adverse reactions. *Journal of Child and Adolescent Psychopharmacology* 2:259–265.

Joseph, J. (2000a). Not in their genes: A critical review of the genetics of attention-deficit hyperactivity disorder. *Developmental Review* 20:539–567.

Joseph, J. (2000b). Problems in psychiatric genetic research: A reply to Faraone and Biederman. *Developmental Review* 20:582–593.

Karch, S. B. (1996). *The Pathology of Drug Abuse,* 2nd ed. Boca Raton, FL: CRC Press.

King, R. A., Riddle, M. A., Chappell, P. B., Hardin, M. T., Anderson, G. M., Lombroso, P., and Scahill, L. (1991, March). Emergence of self-destructive phenomena in children and adolescents during fluoxetine treatment. *Journal of the American Academy of Child and Adolescent Psychiatry* 30:179–186.

Koek, W., and Colpaert, F. C. (1993). Inhibition of methylphenidate-induced behaviors in rats: Differences among neuroleptics. *Journal of Pharmacology and Experimental Therapeutics* 267:181–191.

Lambert, N. (1998). Stimulant treatment as a risk factor for nicotine use and substance abuse. *Program and Abstracts*, pp. 191–8. NIH Consensus Development Conference Diagnosis and Treatment of Attention Deficit Hyperactivity Disorder. November 16–18, 1998, William H. Natcher Conference Center, National Institutes of Health, Bethesda, MD.

Lambert, N., and Hartsough, C. S. (1998). Prospective study of tobacco smoking and substance dependence among samples of ADHD and non-ADHD subjects. *Journal of Learning Disabilities* 31:533–544.

Levine, B. (2001). *Common Sense Rebellion: Debunking Society and Confronting Society.* New York: Continuum.

Lipkin, P. H., Goldstein, I. J., and Adesman, A. R. (1994). Tics and dyskinesias associated with stimulant treatment for attention-deficit hyperactivity disorder. *Archives of Pediatric and Adolescent Medicine* 148:859–861.

Marangell, L., Yudofsky, S., Silver, J. (1999). Psychopharmacology and electroconvulsive therapy. Chapter 27 in Hales, R., Yudofsky, S., and Talbott, J. (eds.). *The American Psychiatric Press Textbook of Psychiatry*, 3rd ed., pp. 1025–1132. Washington, D.C.: American Psychiatric Press.

Marshal, E. (2000, August 4). Duke study faults overuse of stimulants for children. *Science* 289:721.

Maxmen, J. S., and Ward, N. G. (1995). *Psychotropic Drugs Fast Facts,* 2nd ed. New York: W. W. Norton.

Mayes, S. D., Crites, D. L., Bixler, E. O., Humphrey II, F. J., and Mattison, R. E. (1994). Methylphenidate and ADHD: Influence of age, IQ and neurodevelopmental status. *Developmental Medicine and Child Neurology* 36:1099–1107.

Melega, W. P., Raleigh, M. J., Stout, D. B., Huang, S. C., and Phelps, M. E. (1997a). Ethological and 6-[18F]fluoro-L-DOPA-PET profiles of long-term vulnerability to chronic amphetamine. *Behavioural Brain Research* 84:258–268.

Melega, W. P., Raleigh, M. J., Stout, D. B., Lacan, G., Huang, S. C., and Phelps, M. E. (1997b). Recovery of striatal dopamine function after acute amphetamine- and methamphetamine-induced neurotoxicity in the vervet monkey. *Brain Research* 766:113–120.

Morton, C. (2000, November 10). Company, researchers, battle over data access. *Science* 290:1063.

MTA Cooperative Group. (1999a). A 14-month randomized clinical trial of treatment strategies for attention-deficit/hyperactivity disorder. *Archives of General Psychiatry, 56,* 1073–1086.

MTA Cooperative Group. (1999b). Moderators and mediators of treatment response for children with attention-deficit/hyperactivity disorder: The multimodal treatment study of children with attention-deficit hyperactivity disorder. *Archives of General Psychiatry, 56,* 1088–1096.

Nasrallah, H., Loney, J., Olson, S., McCalley-Whitters, M., Kramer, J., and Jacoby, C. (1986). Cortical atrophy in young adults with a history of hyperactivity in childhood. *Psychiatry Research* 17:241–246.

National Toxicology Program. (1995). *NTP Technical Report on Toxicology and Carcinogenesis Studies of Methylphenidate Hydrochloride in F344/N Rats and B6C3F Mice (Feed Studies).* Rockville, MD: National Institutes of Health. NIH Publication No. 95-3355.

Norrholm, S., and Ouimet, C. (2000). Chronic Fluoxetine administration to juvenile rats prevents age-associated dendritic spine proliferation in hippocampus. *Brain Research* 883:205–215.

Oas, P. (2001). *Curing ADD/ADHD Children.* Raleigh, NC: Pentland.

Physicians' Desk Reference. (2001). Montvale, NJ: Medical Economics.

Popper, C. W., and Steingard, R. J. (1994). Disorders usually first diagnosed in infancy, childhood, or adolescence. In R. Hales, S. Yudofsky, and J. Talbott, eds., *The American Psychiatric Press Textbook of Psychiatry,* 2nd ed., pp. 729–832. Washington, D.C.: American Psychiatric Press.

Porrino, L. J., and Lucignani, G. (1987). Different patterns of local brain energy metabolism associated with high and low doses of methylphenidate: Relevance to its action in hyperactive children. *Biological Psychiatry* 22:126–128.

Rapoport, J., Buchsbaum, M., Zahn, T., Weingartner, H., Ludlow, C., and Mikkelsen, E. (1978). Dextroamphetamine: Cognitive and behavior effects in normal prepubertal boys. *Science* 199:560–563.

Richters, J. E., Arnold, L. E., Jensen, P. S., Abikoff, H., Conners, C. K., Greenhill, L. L., Hechtman, L., Hinshaw, S. P., Pelham, W. E., and Swanson, J. M. (1995). NIMH collaborative multisite multimodal treatment study of children with ADHD: I. Background and rationale. *Journal of the American Academy of Child and Adolescent Psychiatry* 34:987–1000.

Riordan, R. M., and Matyas, D. E. (1994, October 11). Letter from legal counsel for CHADD to Thomas A. Constantine, administrator, Drug Enforcement Administration, U.S. Department of Justice. With Attachments. Obtained through Freedom of Information Act (FOIA).

Robinson, T. E., and Kolb, B. (1997). Persistent structural modifications in the nucleus accumbens and prefrontal cortex neurons produced by previous experience with amphetamine. *Journal of Neuroscience* 17:8491–8497.

Rosebush, P., and Mazurek, M. (1999). Neurologic side effects in neuroleptic-naïve patients treated with Haloperidol or Risperidone. *Neurology* 52:782–785.

Sabshin, M. (1992, March 10). To aid understanding of mental disorders. *New York Times.*

Safer, D. J., Allen, R. P., and Barr, E. (1975). Growth rebound after termination of stimulation drugs. *Journal of Pediatrics* 86:113–116.

Sams-Dodd, F., and Newman, J. D. (1997). Effects of administration regime on the psychotomimetic properties of d-amphetamine in the squirrel monkey *(Saimiri sciureus).* *Pharmacology Biochemistry and Behavior* 56:471–480.

Sannerud, C., and Feussner, G. (2000). Is Ritalin an abused drug? Does it meet the criteria for a Schedule II substance? In L. Greenhill and B. Osman, eds., *Ritalin Theory and Practice,* pp. 27–42. New York: Mary Ann Liebert Publishers.

Schteinschnaider, A., Plaghos, L., Garbugino, S., Riveros, D., Lazarowski, A., Intruvini, S., and Massaro, M. (2000). Cerebral arteritis following methylphenidate use. *Journal of Child Neurology* 15:265–267.

Solanto, M. V., and Wender, E. H. (1989). Does methylphenidate constrict cognitive functioning? *Journal of the American Academy of Child and Adolescent Psychiatry* 28:897–902.

Sonsalla, P. K., Jochnowitz, N. D., Zeevalk, G. D., Oostveen, J. A., and Hall, E. D. (1996). Treatment of mice with methamphetamine produces cell loss in the substantia nigra. *Brain Research* 738:172–175.

Spencer, T. J., Biederman, J., Harding, M., O'Donnell D., Faraone, S., and Wilens, T. E. (1996). Growth deficits in ADHD children revisited: Evidence for disorder-associated growth delays? *Journal of the American Academy Child and Adolescent Psychiatry* 35:1460–1469.

Stein, D. (1999). *Ritalin Is Not the Answer.* San Francisco: Jossey-Bass.

Stein, D. (2001). *Unraveling the ADD/ADHD Fiasco.* Kansas City: Andrews McMeel.

Swanson, J. M. (circa 1993). Research synthesis of the effects of stimulant medication on children with attention deficit disorder: A review of reviews. In *Executive Summaries of Research Syntheses and Promising Practices on the Education of Children with Attention Deficit Disorder.* Prepared for Division of Innovation and Development, Office of Special Education Programs, Office of Special Education and Rehabilitation Services, U.S. Department of Education, Washington, D.C. Prepared by the Chesapeake Institute.

Swanson, J. M., Cantwell, D., Lerner, M., McBurnett, K., Pfiffner, L., and Kotkin, R. (1992, Fall). Treatment of ADHD: Beyond medication. *Beyond Behavior* 4 (1):13–16, 18–22.

Thompson, D. (1993, August 19). Financial conflicts of interest in biomedical research. *New England Journal of Medicine* 329:570–576.

Trugman, J. (1988, March 12). Cerebral arteritis and oral methylphenidate. *Lancet* 1:584–585.

University of Buffalo, State University of New York. (2001, November 11). Ritalin may cause long-lasting changes in brain-cell function, UB researchers find. See

www.buffalo.edu/news/fast-execute. . . age.html?article=54330009&hilite
=ritalin.

USA Today (2000, August 15). Editorial: Reading, writing and Ritalin.

Valentine, M. R. (1987). *How to Deal with Discipline Problems in the Schools: A Practical Guide for Educators.* Dubuque, IA: Kendall/Hunt Publishing Company.

Valentine, M. R. (1988). *How to Deal with Difficult Discipline Problems: A Family-Systems Approach.* Dubuque, IA: Kendall/Hunt Publishing Company.

Varley, C., Vincent, J., Varley, P., and Calderon, R. (2001). Emergence of tics in children with attention deficit hyperactivity disorder treated with stimulant medications. *Comprehensive Psychiatry* 42:228–233.

Vastag, B. (2001, August 22/29). Pay attention: Ritalin acts much like cocaine. *Journal of the American Medical Association* 286:905–906.

Volkow, N. D., Ding, Y.-S., Fowler, J. S., Wang, G.-J., Logan, J., Gatley, J. S., Dewey, S., Ashby, C., Lieberman, J., Hitzemann, R., and Wolf, A. P. (1995, June). Is methylphenidate like cocaine? *Archives of General Psychiatry* 52:456–463.

Wang, G.-J., Volkow, N., Fowler, J., Ferrieri, R., Schlyer, D., Alexoff, D., Pappas, N., Lieberman, J., King, P., Warner, D., Wong, C., Hitzemann, R., and Wolf, A. (1994). Methylphenidate decreases regional cerebral blood flow in normal human subjects. *Life Sciences* 54:143–146.

Wegerer, V., Moll, G., Bagli, M., Rothenberger, A., Ruther, E., and Huether G. (1999). Persistently increased density of serotonin transporters in the frontal cortex of rats treated with fluoxetine during early juvenile life. *Journal of Child and Adolescent Psychopharmacology* 9:13–24.

Whalen, C., and Henker, B. (1997). Stimulant pharmacotherapy for attention-deficit/hyperactivity disorders: An analysis of progress, problems, and prospects. In S. Fisher and R. Greenberg, eds., *From Placebo to Panacea: Putting Psychotherapeutic Drugs to the Test*, pp. 323–356. New York: J. Wiley and Sons.

Yudofsky, S., Hales, R., and Ferguson, T. (1991). *What You Need to Know About Psychiatric Drugs.* New York: Grove Weidenfeld.

Zernike, K., and Petersen, M. (2001, August 19). Schools' backing of behavior drugs comes under fire. *New York Times.*

Index

Accommodations for ADHD
    patients, 147–151
Adderall, 1–2, 9, 15, 17–18, 19–20,
    37, 43, 46–47, 54, 58–59,
    62–63, 64, 69, 82
    labeling, 114–117
    XR, 2, 42, 52, 60, 65, 69,
    86–88, 114, 116–117, 207n,
    210n
Adults and ADHD, 135–136
Advertising, drug, 1, 27–29, 88, 96,
    119–120, 124, 195–196, 197,
    213n
Agitation, 17, 32, 75, 82, 93, 95
Alternative treatments, 107–111
*American Dictionary of the English
    Language,* 152
American Psychiatric Association,
    22, 120, 126, 131, 205–206n
American Psychiatric Press, 85, 96
Amitriptyline, 98
Amphetamines. *See* Stimulants
Anafranil, 98
Antacids, 64
Antidepressant Fact Book, The, 94,
    211n, 212n
Antidepressants, 64
    and brain damage, 98–99
    lobotomy-like effects of, 96–98
    use in children, 92–96
Anxiety, 17, 93, 95, 110,
    168–169

Apathy
    and antidepressants, 96–98
    and stimulants, 36–37, 39–40,
    82
Archives of General Psychiatry,
    72–73, 210n
Arteriosclerosis, 64
Attention deficit hyperactivity
    disorder (ADHD)
    accommodating, 147–151
    adult, 135–136
    alternative treatments for,
    107–111
    and brain damage from Ritalin,
    50–51, 83–84, 209–210n
    and brain function, 44–46,
    124–126
    and children under age six, 64–65
    and cocaine use, 50
    compared to physical handicaps,
    147–151
    and conflict resolution, 130–131
    and the Connors Scale, 7
    diagnosing, 6, 22, 28, 93, 110,
    124–136, 147, 161, 166,
    197–200
    as a disability, 147–151
    and drug advertising, 1–2, 28–29
    and drug-impaired attention,
    25–26
    educational alternatives for
    treating, 110–111, 176–188

financial costs of, 199–200
and genetics, 126–129
and malnutrition, 109–110
and mood stabilizers, 106
physical disorders which cause,
109–110, 128
professionals diagnosed with,
148–151
and psychiatric effects of
stimulants, 30–41, 41, 89–91,
211n
and psychosis, 37–39
and Risperdal, 102–103
and Schedule II drugs, 69–72
situational nature of, 131–135,
212n
Aventyl, 98

Baizer, Joan, 48–49
Barkley, Russell, 23
Behavior
and accommodating ADHD
patients, 147–151
and blaming others, 168
and brain function, 122–124
classifying, 126–129
and communication between
parent and child, 166–168
and drug-impaired attention,
25–26, 32–34, 162
drug-induced changes in, 115
and excess energy, 178–180
and fairness, 172–173
hyperactive, 126–129, 178–180
impulsive, 126–129
and individuality of children,
176–181, 182–183,
187–188
and love, 158, 173–174
and moral authority, 155–159,
165, 181, 185–186
and neuroleptics, 102–103
obsessive-compulsive, 20–21, 23,
40, 115

and personal responsibility of
parents, 171–173
problems in school only,
191–192
psychotic, 37–39
reminding children of out-of-
control, 172
and respect, 155–158, 166–167,
185
and sexual abuse, 192, 193
situational nature of, 131–135,
191, 212n
and spontaneity, 20–21, 22
and SSRI-induced lobotomy
syndrome, 96–98
stimulant effects on, 30–41
and stimulants as cause of mental
disorders, 35–40, 161–162
submissive, 19–25
and withdrawal reactions,
68–69, 74–76, 78, 81–83
Benzodiazepines, 105
Beyond Conflict, 213n
Bipolar disorder, 8–9, 93, 106
Blood disorders and stimulants, 62
Brain, the
and antidepressants, 98–99
and blood flow, 44–45
and cognitive toxicity, 32–34
damage from antidepressants,
98–99
damage from Ritalin, 50–51,
83–84
and drug addiction, 71–72
and drug overdose, 44–45
effects of stimulants on, 18–26,
30–41, 43–44, 93–94,
206–207n, 207n
and information processing,
142–143
and the mind, 123
and neuroscience, 122–124
neurotransmitters of, 46–49, 94,
123–124

research on, 26–28
and strokes, 57–59
and supersensitivity to
stimulants, 49–50
and sustained-release stimulants,
52
*Brain-Disabling Treatments in
Psychiatry,* 211n
Breggin, Ginger, 211n
Brookhaven National Laboratory,
44

Caffeine, 41, 82–83
Cardiovascular effects
of antidepressants, 99
of stimulants, 31–32, 33, 53,
56–59, 64, 66
Celexa, 94
CHADD, 70–71
Children
under age six, 64–65, 158–159,
196
and alternative medicine,
107–111
antidepressant use in, 94–99
blaming parents for poisoning,
103–104
and boredom in school, 191–192
brain function of, 45–52,
124–126
cardiovascular problems in,
56–59
and cocaine abuse, 44–45, 48,
49, 50, 72–73
communicating effectively with,
166–168
and conflict resolution, 130–131
and consistency in parenting,
162–164
controlling the authority of,
168–169
and convulsions, 60–61
deemphasizing the value of
conformity in, 201–204

depression and apathy in, 36–37,
39–40, 93, 94–98
diagnosing ADHD in, 6, 22, 28
and discipline, 13–15, 158–159
and drug-impaired attention,
25–26, 32–34, 93–98
drug-induced mania in, 95–96
and drug interactions, 7–12
and drug recalls, 105
educational interventions for,
110–111, 144–146, 176–181
effect of diagnosing ADHD in,
129–131, 166, 183–184,
186–188, 197–200
ending drug use in, 169–170,
188
and excess energy, 178–180
and fairness, 172–173
and growth suppression, 54–56
and home schooling, 192
as individuals, 176–181,
182–183, 187–188
learning disorders in, 137–146
and love, 158, 173–174
malnutrition in, 109–110
and manipulation, 169
measuring intelligence in,
139–140
and mood stabilizing drugs, 106
and moral authority, 153–155,
165, 181
as moral beings, 170–171, 213n
obsessive-compulsive behavior in,
20–21, 23, 40, 93, 206n
and peer abuse, 192, 213n
psychiatric effects of stimulants
on, 22–26, 30–41
psychosis in, 37–39, 207n
and relationships outside the
family, 170
and respect, 155–158, 166–167,
185
and sedatives, 104–105
and self-control, 156

sexual abuse of, 192, 193
of single parents, 164
and situational nature of
    behavior, 131–135, 191, 212n
and SSRI-induced lobotomy
    syndrome, 96–98
strokes in, 57–59
and tardive dyskinesia, 11–12,
    101–102, 205–206n
and the terrorist attacks of
    September 11, 2001, 201–204
and tics, 59–60, 103
who blame others, 168
and withdrawal reactions,
    68–69, 74–84
Cisapride, 99
Citalopram, 94
Clomipramine, 98
Clonazepam, 6
Clonidine, 9, 106
Cocaine, 44–45, 48, 49, 50, 72–73,
    197, 206n
Cognitive toxicity, 32–34
Cohen, David, 11, 79, 106, 211n
Columbine High School, 96
Compazine, 99, 104
Concerta, 1–2, 5, 15, 18, 19–20,
    43, 52, 53, 65, 69, 195, 213n
Conflict resolution, 130–131
Connors Scale, 7
Consensus Development
    Conference on the Diagnosis
    and Treatment of ADHD, 21,
    35–36, 51, 206n
Convulsions and stimulants, 60–61
Cylert, 60, 69

Depakote, 5, 8–9
Department of Education, U.S., 34,
    85–86
Depression
    and antidepressants, 94–98
    and stimulants, 36–37, 39–40,
    64, 118

Desipramine, 98
Desoxyn, 43, 69
Dexedrine, 2, 4, 18, 37, 43, 46–47,
    54, 59, 67, 69, 87, 114
    labeling, 114–116
DextroStat, 69
Diagnosis of attention deficit
    hyperactivity disorder
    (ADHD), 6, 22, 28, 93, 110,
    124–136, 147, 161, 166,
    183–184, 197–200
Diagnostic and Statistical Manual
    of Mental Disorders, IV, 22,
    28, 126, 127, 131–133, 138,
    142
Discipline and behavior, 13–15,
    158–159
Divalproex, 5
Dosage and toxicity, 30–32, 41–42,
    44–45, 71–72, 86–88, 89–91
    and blaming parents for
    poisoning children, 103–104
Doxepin, 98
Drug Enforcement Administration
    (DEA), 69–71, 118, 196,
    210n, 213n
Drugs
    addiction and abuse, 69–73, 105,
    197
    advertising, 1–2, 27–29, 88, 96,
    119–120, 124, 195–196, 197,
    213n
    alternative, 107–111
    antacid, 64
    antidepressant, 64, 92–96
    antipsychotic, 8–11, 34–41,
    92–93, 99–101, 106, 161–162
    and behavior, 19–21
    and blaming parents for
    poisoning children, 103–104
    and brain damage, 46–49
    clinical trials, 35–36, 46–49,
    55–56, 65, 86–89
    and euphoria, 71–72, 118

FDA-approved labeling of, 112–118, 162
and forced submissiveness, 19–25
and growth suppression, 54–56
induced mania, 95–96, 115
interactions, 8–9, 64
lobotomy-like effects of, 96–98
mood stabilizing, 106
overdose, 41–42, 44–45
and the placebo effect, 108
Prozac-like, 94–96
recall of, 105
research, 27–28, 207–208n
schedule II, 69–72, 213n
sedative, 104–105
side effects of, 8–11, 17, 40–41, 114–118
and spontaneity, 20–21
toxicity, 17, 46–49, 100–101
withdrawal symptoms, 12, 78–80, 208–209n. *See also* Stimulants

Educational system
and ADHD, 110–111, 176–181
and boredom in children, 191–192
and children as individuals, 176–181, 182–183
home schooling as an alternative to the traditional, 192, 213n
and learning disorders, 144–146, 176–181
and moral authority, 181, 185–186
parents rights in dealing with the, 193–194
and peer abuse, 192
and school overcrowding, 185
and school recommendations for medical evaluations, 189–194
and teacher stress, 183–186
Effexor, 94
Elavil, 98

Eli Lilly and Company, 96
Ellinwood, Everett, 49
Endocrine and metabolic function and stimulants, 33
Ephedra, 58–59
Euphoria, 71–72, 118
Executive-regulatory functioning, 142–143

Fluoxetine, 94
Fluvoxamine, 94
Focalin, 1–2, 18, 19–20, 43, 69, 82, 205n
Food and Drug Administration (FDA), 2, 10, 11, 17, 27, 30, 31, 47, 58–59, 61, 63, 87, 92, 94, 105, 162
collaboration with drug companies, 119–120
and drug labeling, 112–119, 162, 206–207n, 210n
and Schedule II drugs, 69–72, 213n

Gastrointestinal system
and neuroleptic drugs, 99–100, 104
and stimulants, 33, 61
Genetics and ADHD, 126–129
Geodon, 99, 162
Glaucoma, 64
Goddard, Ian, 212n
Good Housekeeping, 1
Growth suppression and stimulants, 54–56

Hair loss and pulling and stimulants, 61
Haldol, 11, 60, 99, 103, 162
Hallucinations, 6, 10, 32, 66
Harris, Eric, 96, 211n
Harvard Medical School, 48
Headaches and stimulants, 61, 66, 82

Head injuries, 110, 128
Heart of Being Helpful, The, 154,
    213n
Home schooling, 192
Hospitalization for withdrawal
    symptoms, 79–80
Hyperactivity, 126–129, 134,
    178–180
Hypertension, 64, 106
Hyperthyroidism, 64
Hypoglycemia, 110

Imipramine, 98
Impulsivity, 126–129, 134
    in parents, 167
Individuality of children, 176–181,
    182–183, 187–188
Insomnia, 17, 93, 94, 104–105
Intelligence quotient (IQ), 139–140,
    212n
International Center for the Study
    of Psychiatry and Psychology,
    212–213n
Irritability, 17, 75, 110, 125

Jensen, Peter, 21–22, 39, 89
Journal of Child and Adolescent
    Psychopharmacology, 97
Journal of Child Neurology, 58
Journal of the American Medical
    Association, 43, 213n

Klonopin, 6, 8, 9, 93, 105

Ladies' Home Journal, 1
Lancet, 58
Lead poisoning, 110, 128
Learning disorders (LD)
    and bright children, 141–142
    diagnosing, 137–139
    and information processing,
        142–143
    and IQ, 139–140, 212n
    parents guidelines for assessing,
        190–191

    psychiatric drug treatment for,
        143
    and reversing letters, 141
Liver tumors and stimulants, 63
Lobotomy-like effects of SSRIs,
    96–98
Long-term effects of stimulant use,
    85–91
Luvox, 94, 96, 211n

Malnutrition, 109–110
Manic-depression, 8, 92–93, 95,
    106
McNeil Consumer Health Care,
    195–196, 213n
Mellaril, 11, 60, 162
Metadate, 2, 52, 53, 65, 69, 195
Methylin SR, 52, 69
Metoclopramide, 99
Midazolam, 105
Monoamine oxidase inhibitors
    (MAOIs), 64
Mood stabilizers, 106
Mood swings, 8, 207n
Moral authority and behavior,
    153–155, 165, 181, 185–186
Munchausen's by Proxy, 103

Nardil, 64
National Institute of Mental Health
    (NIMH), 9–10, 45, 65, 74, 85,
    88–89
National Institutes of Health (NIH),
    21, 35
National Toxicology Program, 210n
Navane, 11
Neuroleptics, 8–11, 99–100
    malignant syndrome (NMS), 63,
        100
    and tardive dyskinesia, 11–12,
        101–102, 205–206n
    and tics, 103
Neuroscience, 122–124
Neurotransmitters, 46–49, 94,
    123–124

New England Journal of Medicine,
120
New York Times, 120
Noritriptyline, 98
Norpramin, 98
Novartis, 2, 69–70, 205n

Obsessive-compulsive behaviors,
20–21, 23, 40, 93, 115
Olanzapine, 99
Orap, 103
Overdose, stimulant, 30–32, 41–42,
44–45, 71–72, 86–88, 89–91
and blaming parents for
poisoning children, 103–104

Pamelor, 98
Parents and caregivers
avoiding anger, 167, 173
and childrens' relationships
outside the family, 170
and children who blame others,
168
and communicating authority,
154–155, 165–166
communication skills for,
166–168
controlling the authority of
children, 168–169
and deemphasizing the value of
conformity among children,
201–204
developing consistency between,
162–164
and discipline, 13–15, 158–159
and fairness, 172–173
guidelines for dealing with school
recommendations, 189–194
guidelines for regaining control
of family life, 165–169,
212–213n
and love, 158, 173–174
manipulation by children, 169
moral authority of, 153–154,
165, 198–199

and respect, 155–158
rights of, 154, 193–194
seeking professional help,
159–160
single, 164
taking personal responsibility,
171–173
and the terrorist attacks of
September 11, 2001, 201–204
viewing children as moral beings,
170–171
Parnate, 64
Paroxetine, 94
Paxil, 94
Pediatrics, 36
Peer abuse, 192, 213n
Pemoline, 60, 69
Phenergan, 104
Physicians' Desk Reference, 17, 64,
95, 106, 112–113, 115,
116–117, 118, 207n, 210n
Placebo effects of treatments, 108,
212n
Preexisting conditions and
stimulants, 64
Pregnancy, nursing and stimulants,
62–63
Prochlorperazine, 99
Prolixin, 11
Propulsid, 99, 104
Prostatic hypertrophy, 64
Prozac-like antidepressants, 94–99,
211n
*Psychiatric Drugs: Hazards to the
Brain,* 114
Psychiatry, 4–5, 125–126
case study, 5–15
damage to children from,
186–188
and misinformation, 112–120,
211–212n
prescribing of drugs in, 34–41,
89, 92–94, 106, 143, 190, 200
and stimulant withdrawal,
78–80

Psychological effects of diagnosing
  ADHD, 129–131, 197–200
Psychosis, 37–39, 89–91, 92, 95,
  118, 207n
  drug-induced, 115

Quetiapine, 11, 99

Rather, Dan, 205–206n
Reclaiming Our Children, 188,
  212n
Reglan, 99, 104
Religion, 202–203
Respect and behavior, 155–158,
  166–167, 185
Risperdal, 6, 9–10, 11–12, 15, 60,
  99, 102–103, 162
Ritalin, 65
  abuse potential of, 69–70
  backlash against, 195–196
  behavior effects of, 7–11, 15,
    19–21, 36–37
  and blood disorders, 62
  brain effect of, 43, 50–51
  cardiovascular effects of, 57
  and cocaine abuse, 44–45, 48,
    49, 50, 72–73
  and cognitive toxicity, 33–34
  contraindications to, 17–18
  and depression and apathy,
    36–37
  dosage increases, 7–8
  and drug advertising, 1–2,
    195–196
  and drug interactions, 8–9, 11
  early use of, 4
  effect on brain of, 44–46, 47–49,
    209n
  and ephedra, 58–59
  and the gastrointestinal system,
    33, 61
  LA, 2, 69
  and liver tumors, 63
  and neuroleptic malignant
    syndrome (NMS), 63

and preexisting conditions, 64
pressure to prescribe, 4–5, 89–91
principles of withdrawal from,
    78–80
and psychosis, 37–39
as a Schedule II drug, 69–72
side effects of, 17–18, 30, 32–34,
    118
similarity to cocaine of, 44–45
SR, 52, 65, 69, 87
and strokes, 57–59
and tics, 59–60
toxicity, 17–18, 47–49, 75–76,
    209–210n
use in children under age six,
    64–65
and withdrawal reactions, 67–69.
    See also Stimulants
Roche Laboratories, 105
Rolaids, 64

Schedule II drugs, 69–72, 213n
Schizophrenia, 6, 9–10, 92
Science, 210n
Sedatives, 104–105
Seizures, 60–61, 110
Serax, 105
Seroquel, 11, 99, 162
Sertraline, 94
Sexual abuse, 192, 193
Sexual dysfunction and stimulants,
    62
Shire US Inc., 37, 114, 195, 212n
Sinequan, 99
Skin and joint disorders and
    stimulants, 62, 118
SmithKline Beecham, 114
Society for Neuroscientists, 48
Spontaneity, 20–21, 22
SSRI-induced lobotomy syndrome,
    96–98
Stimulants
  and apathy, 36–37, 39–40, 82
  backlash against, 195–196
  and behavior, 19–21, 32–34

behavior effects of, 16–18,
22–26, 28–29
and blood disorders, 62
and blurred vision, 61
and the brain, 18–21, 30–34,
46–49
cardiovascular effects of, 31–32,
33, 53, 56–59, 64, 66
as cause of mental disorders,
35–40
clinical trials, 35–36, 46–49,
55–56, 65, 86–89
and cocaine abuse, 44–45, 48,
49, 50, 72–73, 197, 206n
and convulsions, 60–61
and depression, 36–37, 39–40,
64, 118
dosage, 30–32, 41–42, 44–45,
71–72, 89–91
and drug labeling, 112–118,
206–207n, 210n
effects on the body, 54–66,
114–118, 205–206n
effects on the brain, 49–52,
206–207n, 207n
and endocrine and metabolic
function, 33
and ephedra, 58–59
and euphoria, 71–72, 118
and the gastrointestinal system,
33, 61
and growth suppression, 54–56
guidelines for withdrawal from,
78–80
and hair loss and pulling, 61
and headaches, 61, 66, 82
interactions with other drugs, 64
and liver tumors, 63
long-term effects of using,
85–91
and obsessive-compulsive
behaviors, 20–21, 23, 40,
206n
and overstimulation of children,
17–18, 206n

and preexisting conditions, 64
and pregnancy and nursing,
62–63
prevalence of use, 196–197,
213n
psychiatric effects of, 30–34,
114–118
and psychosis, 37–39
Schedule II, 69–72, 213n
and seizures, 60–61
and sexual dysfunction, 62
and skin and joint disorders, 62
and strokes, 57–59
supersensitivity to, 49–50
sustained-release, 52, 65–66
and tics, 59–60, 209n
toxicity, 17–18, 30–34, 42,
209–210n
use in children under age six,
64–65, 196
withdrawal and rebound
reactions to, 33, 63, 74–84,
208–209n
zombie effect of, 34, 39–40. *See
also* Ritalin
Strokes, 57–59
Submissiveness, forced, 19–25
Suicide, 40
Supersensitivity to stimulants,
49–50
Sustained-release stimulants, 52,
65–66
Swanson, James, 51

Talking Back to Prozac, 211n
Talking Back to Ritalin, 5, 36, 46,
71, 89, 120, 124, 206n, 211n,
212n, 213n
Tardive dyskinesia, 11–12,
101–102, 205–206n
Ten-percent-per-week guideline,
80
Terrorist attacks of September 11,
2001, 201–204
Textbook of Psychiatry, 85, 96

Thorazine, 11
Tics
    and antidepressants, 98
    and neuroleptics, 103
    and stimulants, 59–60, 209n
Tourette's disorder, 10, 103
Toxicity of stimulants, 17–18,
    30–34, 42, 46–49, 75–76,
    209–210n
Toxic Psychiatry, 120, 207–208n,
    211n
Tranquilizers, 104–105
Tricyclics, 98–99
Tums, 64

Underachievers, 137–139
University of Pittsburgh, 95

Valium, 105
Venlafaxine, 94
Versed, 105
Violence, 17, 32
Vision and stimulants, 61

War Against Children of Color,
    The, 212n
Washington Post, 58–59
Webster, Noah, 152

Western Psychiatric Institute and
    Clinic, 34
Withdrawal and rebound reactions
    to stimulants, 33, 63, 68–69,
    74–76, 208–209n
    and caffeine, 82–83
    and label warnings, 67–68
    permanent symptoms of, 83–84
    physical basis of, 81–82
    positive reinforcements to
        counter, 80–81
    principles of, 78–80
    and the ten-percent-per-week
        guideline, 80

Xanax, 105

Yale University, 95
Your Drug May Be Your Problem:
    How and Why to Stop Taking
    Psychiatric Medications, 11,
    79, 105, 106, 211n

Ziprasidone, 99
Zoloft, 94
Zombie effect of stimulants, 34,
    39–40
Zyprexa, 11, 99, 162

About the Author

Peter R. Breggin, M.D., has been in the full-time private practice of psychiatry in Bethesda, Maryland, and the Washington, D.C., area since 1968. He treats adults, children, and families.

Dr. Breggin is a well-known critic of biological psychiatry, including medication, and a strong advocate for psychological and social human services. He is founder and Director Emeritus of the International Center for the Study of Psychiatry and Psychology (ICSPP), a nonprofit organization of nearly 2,000 reform-minded professionals that has been called "the conscience of psychiatry." He is founder and former editor-in-chief of the peer-review professional journal *Ethical Human Sciences and Services*.

Dr. Breggin is the author of many professional articles and numerous books, including *Toxic Psychiatry* (1991), *Talking Back to Prozac* (with his wife, Ginger Breggin, 1994), *The War Against Children of Color* (with Ginger Breggin, 1998), *Your Drug May Be Your Problem: How and Why to Stop Taking Psychiatric Medications* (with David Cohen, 1999), *Reclaiming Our Children: A Healing Solution for a Nation in Crisis* (2000), *Talking Back to Ritalin* (revised, 2001), and *The Antidepressant Fact Book* (2001).

Dr. Breggin was trained at Harvard College and Case Western Reserve Medical School. His residency in psychiatry was at the Massachusetts Mental Health Center and at the State University of New York, Upstate Medical Center. He is a former full-time consultant with the National Institute of Mental Health (NIMH) and has held teaching appointments at Harvard Medical School, the Washington School of Psychiatry, George Mason University, and the Johns Hopkins University Department of Counseling. He was selected by the National Institutes of Health (NIH) as the scientific expert on psychiatric drugs and their adverse effects on children at the NIH Consensus Development Conference on the Diagnosis and Treatment of Attention Deficit Hyperactivity Disorder.

Dr. Breggin has participated as a medical expert in a variety of criminal and civil legal cases involving the harmful effects of psychiatric drugs, constitutional rights of patients, malpractice, and product liability. He formulated the scientific basis for dozens of continuing product liability suits brought against Eli Lilly and Co. concerning Prozac-induced violence and suicide. His work inspired the recent class-action suits brought against Novartis, the manufacturer of Ritalin, for conspiring with the American Psychiatric Association to overinflate the value and use of the ADHD diagnosis and stimulants.

Dr. Breggin's views are regularly covered in the national media, including the *New York Times, Washington Post, Time, Newsweek, USA Today, People Magazine, 60 Minutes, 20/20,* and *Nightline.*

More about Dr. Breggin and his work—including a complete résumé—can be found on his web site, www.breggin.com.